ZONE
MEALS
IN
SECONDS

Also by Dr. Barry Sears

The Zone

Mastering the Zone

Zone Food Blocks

Zone-Perfect Meals in Minutes

The Top 100 Zone Foods

A Week in the Zone

The Soy Zone

The Omega Rx Zone

What to Eat in the Zone

ZONE

MEALS

IN

SECONDS

150 Fast and Delicious Recipes for
Breakfast, Lunch, and Dinner

Dr. Barry Sears and Lynn Sears

ReganBooks
An Imprint of HarperCollinsPublishers

ZONE MEALS IN SECONDS. Copyright © 2004 by Dr. Barry Sears and Lynn Sears. All rights reserved. Printed in the United States of America. No part of this book may be used or reproduced in any manner whatsoever without written permission except in the case of brief quotations embodied in critical articles and reviews. For information address HarperCollins Publishers Inc., 10 East 53rd Street, New York, NY 10022.

HarperCollins books may be purchased for educational, business, or sales promotional use. For information please write: Special Markets Department, HarperCollins Publishers Inc., 10 East 53rd Street, New York, NY 10022.

FIRST EDITION

Designed by Nancy Singer Olaguera

Library of Congress Cataloging-in-Publication Data
Sears, Barry, 1947–
    Zone meals in seconds : 150 fast and delicious recipes for breakfast, lunch, and dinner / Barry Sears and Lynn Sears.—1st ed.
      p. cm.
    Includes index.
    ISBN 0-06-039311-4
    1. Reducing diets. 2. Reducing diets—Recipes. 3. Nutrition. I. Sears, Lynn. II. Title.
RM222.2.S3924 2004
641.5'635—dc22
                                                                 2003066684

04 05 06 07 08 ❖/RRD 10 9 8 7 6 5 4 3 2

To our daughters, Kelly and Kristin,
the first children to enter the Zone

Contents

Acknowledgments

We would like to thank Cris Jochum and Monica Trindade for reading early drafts of this book and for their words of encouragement. We appreciate the diverse recipes submitted by Rachel Albert-Matesz and Diane Manteca. We'd also like to thank our team at ReaganBooks, particularly Cassie Jones for her excellent final editing of this book. As always, our greatest thanks go to Judith Regan for her courage and foresight to support and publish the Zone concepts.

Introduction

My husband, Barry Sears, often says that any fool can eat one cup of pasta at a meal, but it's much harder to eat twelve cups of broccoli. I'd like to add to that statement. No fool would ever want to chop twelve cups of broccoli for one meal.

When you're in the Zone, you will eat lots of vegetables and fruit, plus a moderate amount of low-fat protein and a dash of monounsaturated fat. In just a few days you'll feel more energetic, have more mental focus, and begin to notice that your clothes fit better. So why would anyone decide not to live in the Zone for a lifetime?

I'm afraid that some people think the Zone is too complicated and requires lots of chopping and chomping of vegetables, but it's really not complicated. Meal preparation is a snap in the Zone, and, no, you won't have to chop twelve cups of broccoli for dinner. The lifestyle called the Zone dietary program is simple to master.

Of course, my favorite type of meal preparation is getting dressed to go out to dinner. On other nights I am the person who has to prepare dinners under the watchful eyes of my husband, Dr. Barry Sears, the creator of the Zone diet. Lucky me. Fortunately, I'm no fool. I've learned plenty of simple tricks to make Zone meal preparation a snap, and I'll share them with you in this book.

In fact, I'll go far beyond tricks for preparing breakfast, lunch, and dinner at home. The real Zone challenge begins when you leave your front door and need to figure out what to eat for lunch during the workday in an office surrounded by fast-food joints and vending machines. I've been a newspaper reporter and editor for many years. My husband's observation years ago after visiting my newspaper office was that most editors and reporters end up looking like Ed Asner of *Lou Grant* and *The Mary Tyler Moore Show.* Although some of my brothers and sisters in journalism have avoided that fate, many more have not.

Think about it. Reporters find their stories and then come back to the newspaper's offices, sit down, and write. Editors sit while they edit the stories. Often, when they're facing a particularly tight deadline, they eat lunches and dinners while writing and editing. And what do reporters and editors eat? They eat stuff from the vending machine: Fritos, Twizzlers, candy bars. Then they wash it all down with a soda. Deadlines always cause feeding frenzies. One copy editor friend of mine has a favorite snack. He opens a can of Coke, uses a Twizzler as a straw, and then eats the Twizzler after he finishes the Coke.

Reporters and editors who have more time get take-out food, and lots of it: ziti and meatballs, calzones, pizzas, subs and french fries, doughnuts, chinese food with plenty of fried rice. When I last worked in a newspaper office two years ago, even I, the first lady of the Zone, after years of being happily in the Zone, began to see the pounds start to slowly pile on. Fortunately, my husband quickly took notice, and that was the end of that. I returned to the Zone, and the pounds slid off.

In *Zone Meals in Seconds,* you'll learn how to avoid the fast-food lunch trap. We'll also tell you how to survive cocktail parties, holiday parties, buffets, barbecues, dining out, and just about every culinary experience there is. Chapter 8, "The Can-Do Zone," shows you how to open a couple of cans and use frozen food to create meals in minutes. Chapter 9, "Slow Cooking in the Zone," tells you how to cook meals overnight, ready to take to work for lunch the next day, or cook your meals during the day so that dinner will be ready when you come home.

Even finicky kids can live happily in the Zone. We've raised two of our own and have learned every trick in the book. When our older daughter reached her early teens, she became a vegetarian, which presented an interesting dietary dilemma. We'll show you how we helped her stay in the Zone while adhering to her vegetarian diet. Our younger daughter was a very picky eater. One very wearisome year she ate grilled chicken over lettuce with grapes and Granny Smith apples for dinner just about every night. I'm surprised she didn't turn green, but at least that dinner kept her in the Zone. Happily, she outgrew her monotonous diet and now eats a wide variety of Zone foods.

No matter what your cooking style—from purist to Where's the can opener?—I hope you'll discover through this book how to painlessly stay in the Zone.

Many of these recipes have been created by Rachel Albert-Matesz, a freelance food and health writer, cooking coach, and natural foods cooking instructor who lives in Phoenix, Arizona. Her forthcoming book, *The Garden of Eating: A Produce-Dominated Diet and Cookbook,* will be published in early 2004. You can definitely call her a purist.

Diane Manteca provided the recipes for chapter 8. Her recipes will help people who want to use prepared foods to cut down the amount of time needed to make meals. A chef and the owner of the Brickyard Café, a wonderfully eclectic restaurant in Cambridge, Massachusetts, Diane has been involved in the food business for sixteen years and has taught cooking for nine years. Prior to branching out with her own business, Diane was a chef at Formaggio Kitchen in Cambridge and L'Alouette in Lexington, Massachusetts.

And what is my cooking style? I'm not even sure you can call it a style, but I've learned how to create simple and tasty Zone meals that please my family and me. I'll also share my own story with you. In my pre-Zone days I tried every diet known to womankind—and failed every diet known to womankind. Maybe you can relate.

My dietary quest ended when I entered the Zone. The Zone works. I can attest to that. People say it's easy for me to say that because I'm naturally thin. I reply that I am certainly not naturally thin. My trip back to a newsroom about two years ago proved to me that I could very easily get naturally fat again. One thing has to be made clear from the start: The Zone is not a dietary plan you'll follow for a few weeks or a few months, lose weight, and then go back to eating as you used to do. You will practice the Zone lifestyle for the rest of your long, healthy, slim life. I hope this book will make the Zone way of life easier to achieve than ever before.

What are the rewards of the Zone lifestyle? For one thing, you'll easily slip into a single-digit dress and slacks size. For another, you won't need to pick up *Family Circle, Woman's Day* or other magazines at the grocery check-out counter every week. You may have noticed that the cover of these magazines usually includes two features. The first is the proclamation of a new diet nestled inside the magazine that will be the last diet you'll ever need—the diet to end all diets. The second is a picture of a delicious-looking cake or pie (recipe inside). In my pre-Zone days, I'd buy a magazine about every other week and try the featured diet. After about a day and a half, I'd be so famished and light-headed that I'd abandon the diet and make the cake or pie recipe instead.

The absolute worst diet I ever tried lasted exactly two meals. For breakfast, I was told to have coffee and half a grapefruit. For lunch I had "all the fruit salad you want." At dinner, near starvation and about ready to faint due to low blood sugar from consuming all carbohydrates and no protein at all, I ate everything and anything I wanted. I was through with that diet.

Although I was slender when I got married, I should have looked a generation back at my mother, who began to gain weight when she was in her thirties and just kept on going. My mother was northern Italian, and she and her sisters suffered from a tendency toward Renaissance flesh, or as it was more commonly referred to around the family dining room table, the Bruno build. When I was married, I weighed 123 pounds. By age forty, at 5 feet, 5½ inches, I weighed 156 pounds. I was beginning to resign myself to a life spent wearing A-line skirts and blazers or muumuus and bathing suits with skirts when the weather was hotter. At size fourteen, I looked and felt dumpy.

I also began to feel light-headed between meals, especially when I was following the latest fad diet. I had every medical test on the books, but the doctors found nothing wrong. One arrogant male doctor looked down his nose at me and said that with two small children and a newspaper job, I was obviously having anxiety attacks. Great, I thought. He thinks I'm just another neurotic housewife. The more I thought about it, the more I thought his diagnosis was wrong. I didn't feel anxious, just light-headed and shaky.

Then I made my own diagnosis. I was sure I had hypoglycemia. I hit on this idea when I thought back to my mother's eating habits when I was growing up. She constantly said, "I feel shaky and I have to eat something now." And she was constantly eating. When I asked my doctor to be tested for hypoglycemia, he replied, "There is no such thing as hypoglycemia. It's all in your mind." That was back in 1982, and I certainly hope no doctor would make that statement today.

Our family meals when I was growing up weren't that far off the Zone mark, especially in comparison to today's lamentable grain-laden dietary standards. We'd eat meat or fish and vegetables and a salad for dinner, but dinner was always accompanied by a starch—mashed potatoes (my father's favorite), rice, or pasta. A basket of dinner rolls usually sat on the table. And my mother's favorite snack was popcorn—lots of popcorn every night before she went to bed and on Sunday afternoons while she and Dad watched the Bears, Bulls, or Cubs games. As you read this book, you'll understand why she had those shaky feelings, and why I did, too.

I was not the only one gaining weight. Barry was, too, even though he had been a very active athlete. For my husband the stakes were particularly high. The men in his family had an unfortunate penchant for dying of heart disease in their early fifties. Beginning in about 1980, when the weight started to pile on, Barry and I tried everything. We experimented with high-carbohydrate diets, high-protein diets, and even a liquid diet. Nothing worked. Arriving at the Zone didn't happen overnight. Until about 1988, I cooked much as my mother did. We had eggs, toast, and cereal for breakfast (a meal I often skipped), a sandwich and maybe soup for lunch, and some sort of protein (probably much more than what is recommended in the Zone), a vegetable, and a starch for dinner. By ten o'clock at night, Barry and I would be rummaging around the kitchen for something to eat. Usually junk food.

Barry began to devote a great deal of his research time trying to discover a dietary plan that would both treat my hypoglycemia and avert his own family history of premature heart disease. Finally, he found a research article written back in 1985 in the *New England Journal of Medicine* ("Paleolithic nutrition: A consideration of its nature and current implications," S.B. Eaton, M. Konner, 312:283–289, January 31, 1985) that described what our earliest ancestors ate. What was the diet of the caveman? Lean protein, vegetables, and fruit.

Barry's first suggestion in that banner year, 1988, was that every meal we ate at home should include protein, and I should replace the starch portion of dinner (potatoes, pasta, rice, and/or bread) with additional vegetables, or perhaps some fruit for dessert. At first, I thought removing the starch would deprive my family and carry the perception that I was lazy, but I tried it. Amazingly, even if I removed the starch and didn't add more vegetables or fruit, we were no longer going into a feeding frenzy at bedtime. Less was indeed more. If we were hungry later in the evening, we ate a bit of cheese (protein) and fruit (carbohydrate). The cravings for junk food diminished, and we began to lose weight and feel more energetic. Most important, my so-called anxiety attacks were gone. Long before the publication of *The Zone* in 1995, Barry continued to refine his dietary program, and I tried to adapt his research in what can basically be called the first Zone test kitchen. Again, lucky me.

My husband likes to talk about eicosanoids and about treating food as if it is a drug. You know what? I'm not going to go there. If you want the scientific principles behind the Zone—and believe me, the dietary plan is based on cutting-edge science—then start with *A Week in the Zone.* Matriculate to *Mastering the Zone.* Get your Zone bachelor's degree by reading *The Zone,* and if you want to get your master's, venture into *The Anti-Aging Zone* and *The OmegaRx Zone. Zone-Perfect Meals in Minutes* contains a lot of great recipes. And vegetarians and other people who want to add soy to their diets will enjoy *The Soy Zone.*

All you need to know about the science of the Zone right now is what I needed to know to start eating correctly. The Zone philosophy centers on keeping the hormone insulin within a Zone, not too high and not too low. You need some insulin to live because it drives nutrients to your cells, but too much insulin creates a health nightmare. Excess insulin makes you fat, accelerates heart disease, and shortens your life span.

When you stop controlling insulin, all hell breaks loose. Perhaps that's why there's an epidemic of obesity and type-2 diabetes in this country, both conditions caused by excess insulin production. The likely cause of this obesity epidemic is the emphasis the government places on starchy carbohydrates, which when eaten with wild abandon, make insulin levels rise sky high, with the corresponding low blood sugar. That leads to feelings of light-headedness and hunger. What happens then? You reach for a high-carbohydrate snack, which temporarily lifts you up before dropping you down with a thud back into carbohydrate hell.

Now you know why my popcorn-loving mother had to keep eating more carbohydrates to keep her energy up. Not all carbohydrates have this adverse impact. Most vegetables and fruits, such as berries, don't cause an insulin spike.

So let's get started. Take it from me, it's a great feeling to finally find an eating plan that is so easy to follow. Being in the Zone brings a wonderful sense of freedom because you know you'll never have to pick up another magazine that promises a miracle diet.

—*Lynn Sears*

Getting Started

The Zone Diet wasn't created overnight. We took baby steps as we began to walk to the center of the Zone. Remember that the first thing we did was to eliminate starch from our meals. We noticed an immediate improvement. We were no longer hungry at bedtime, and if we were, we would eat a piece of cheese (protein and fat) and some fruit (carbohydrate). This chapter will allow you to enter the Zone at several different levels as well. Many of you reading this book have already read other Zone books, and are reading this one for new tips and recipes. Others may be Zone experts. Still others may be learning about the Zone for the first time. Jump in where you feel comfortable.

LEVEL ONE: As you read this book and begin to understand its principles, we hope you will immediately begin to substitute vegetables and fruits for much of the bread, pasta, rice, and potatoes that you eat. Not all fruits and vegetables are created equal because some raise insulin levels more than others do. Vegetables to avoid or use in moderation include carrots, corn, and beets. Fruits to avoid or use in moderation include raisins, most tropical fruits, cranberries, and bananas. Berries are the most Zone-favorable fruit. A complete Zone Food Block Guide, listing favorable and unfavorable protein, carbohydrate, and fat choices is found on page 365.

Use what we call the hand-eye method. Divide your plate into thirds. On one-third, place low-fat protein, such as chicken, fish, egg whites, cottage cheese, or soy products. The portion should be the size and depth of the palm of your hand. Fill the other two-thirds with vegetables and fruit. After your plate is full, add a dash of fat, such as olive oil, avocado, or nuts.

You should eat three meals and two snacks every day. For meals use a dinner plate, and for snacks use a dessert plate. Use this little ditty to help you understand which foods are protein and which are carbohydrates: "Carbohydrates grow in the ground, and protein (with the exception of soy) moves around." Make sure you drink lots of water and avoid caffeine and soda as much as possible.

Now, learn the Zoning by-laws. Timing is important. Make sure to eat breakfast within one hour of waking. Don't ever let more than four to five hours go by before eating lunch. Have a snack either mid-morning or mid-afternoon. The timing of this snack depends upon the length of time between either breakfast and lunch or lunch and dinner. For example, you might eat breakfast at 8 A.M. and lunch at noon. Dinner might not come until 7 P.M., which means you'll need a small snack at 4 or 5 P.M. On the other hand, you may eat breakfast at 6 A.M. and not have time for lunch until 1 P.M. In that case have your snack in the mid-morning. Remember, you don't want to let more than five hours go by before your next meal or snack. Use the same hand-eye approach that you use to construct your Zone meals, except use a dessert-size plate to construct your snack. (Check out a list of snack ideas in chapter 6.)

The wonderful thing about the Zone dietary program is that you will never be hungry because your blood sugar is stable. If the brain isn't hungry, then you won't feel hungry. You will never go more than four or five hours without eating, except when you go to bed. And before you go to bed, make sure you end your day with a Zone snack. Remember, even if you are asleep, your brain is still working. A favorite bedtime snack is 1 ounce of cheese and a glass of wine. (Treat alcohol as a carbohydrate.)

To help with the planning, here are a few examples for your first day in the center of the Zone. You'll read many other suggestions in the chapters on breakfasts, lunches, and dinners. This first breakfast suggestion shows how substantial a meal can be on the Zone diet.

BREAKFAST FOR WOMEN (should be eaten within one hour of waking):

Omelet made with ½ cup egg substitute, 1 ounce low-fat cheese (feta is great), a couple of sun-dried tomatoes, chopped, and a bit of chopped basil

⅔ cup slow-cooking oatmeal sprinkled with cinnamon and 3 macadamia nuts, crushed

1 cup raspberries (fresh or frozen)

BREAKFAST FOR MEN (should be eaten within one hour of waking):

Omelet made with ¾ cup egg substitute, 1 ounce low-fat cheese, a couple of sun-dried tomatoes, chopped, and a bit of chopped basil

1 cup slow-cooking oatmeal sprinkled with cinnamon and 4 macadamia nuts, crushed

1 cup raspberries (fresh or frozen)

For people who begin their day with a trip to the gym, here's a simple breakfast to eat before you go.

FOR WOMEN:

Blend the following in a blender. Add ice, if desired.

21 grams protein powder

1½ cups frozen blueberries, defrosted

3 teaspoons slivered almonds

FOR MEN:

> 28 grams protein powder
>
> 2 cups frozen blueberries, defrosted
>
> 4 teaspoons slivered almonds

Still too hard? Try this.

FOR WOMEN:

> 1 ounce low-fat cheese
>
> 1 Wasa cracker
>
> ½ cup low-fat cottage cheese
>
> 6 cashews
>
> ⅔ cup unsweetened applesauce

Melt the low-fat cheese on the cracker. Mix the cottage cheese, cashews, and applesauce together or eat them however you like.

FOR MEN:

> 1 ounce low-fat cheese
>
> 1 Wasa cracker
>
> ¾ cup low-fat cottage cheese
>
> 8 cashews
>
> 1 cup unsweetened applesauce

Melt the low-fat cheese on the cracker. Mix the cottage cheese, cashews, and applesauce together or eat however you like.

If you don't like any of these choices, go directly to chapter 3 and pick out a winning breakfast combination for your first day in the Zone, or try some of Rachel's breakfast recipes, also in chapter 3.

LUNCH FOR WOMEN:

3 ounces cooked skinless chicken breast strips on lettuce leaves

Olive oil and vinegar dressing (1 teaspoon olive oil plus vinegar, salt, and pepper to taste)

1 apple

1 small breadstick

LUNCH FOR MEN:

4 ounces cooked skinless chicken breast on lettuce leaves

Olive oil and vinegar dressing (1⅓ teaspoons olive oil plus vinegar, salt, and pepper to taste)

1 apple

½ cup grapes

1 small breadstick

FOR WOMEN:

Mix together

¾ cup low-fat cottage cheese

½ cup chickpeas

¼ cup kidney beans

3 macadamia nuts, crushed

FOR MEN:

Mix together

1 cup low-fat cottage cheese

½ cup chickpeas

½ cup kidney beans

4 macadamia nuts, crushed

FOR WOMEN:

Chili made from

3 ounces ground turkey

½ cup salsa

¼ cup black beans

1 ounce grated low-fat cheese sprinkled on top

½ orange for dessert

FOR MEN:

Chili made from

4½ ounces ground turkey

½ cup salsa

½ cup black beans

1 ounce grated low-fat cheese sprinkled on top

½ orange for dessert

You may want to check out the suggested combinations in chapter 4 for other simple Zone lunches. Or try Rachel's lunch recipes in chapter 4 and Diane's recipes in chapter 8.

DINNER FOR WOMEN:

3 ounces cooked skinless chicken breast

1 small salad containing 1 cup canned artichoke hearts, drained, with a dressing of 1 teaspoon olive oil plus vinegar to taste

2 cups cooked zucchini

½ cup seedless grapes

DINNER FOR MEN:

4 ounces cooked skinless chicken breast

1 small salad containing 1 cup canned artichoke hearts with a dressing of 1⅓ teaspoons olive oil plus vinegar to taste

2 cups cooked zucchini

1 cup seedless grapes

FOR WOMEN:

4½ ounces grilled salmon

1½ cups green beans mixed with

3 macadamia nuts, crushed

1 apple for dessert

FOR MEN:

6 ounces grilled salmon

1½ cups green beans mixed with

4 macadamia nuts, crushed

Fruit salad of

⅓ cup Mandarin oranges packed in water

and 1 sliced apple

FOR WOMEN:

1 soy burger

1 ounce low-fat cheese

¼ cup chickpeas

¼ cup kidney beans

¼ cup black beans

Mix the beans with a vinaigrette of 1 teaspoon olive oil plus vinegar to taste.

FOR MEN:

1 soy burger

2 ounces low-fat cheese

½ cup chickpeas

¼ cup kidney beans

¼ cup black beans

1 peach

Mix the beans with a vinaigrette of 1⅓ teaspoons olive oil plus vinegar to taste.

Chapter 5 contains a number of other simple dinner combinations or check out Rachel's dinner recipes, also in chapter 5, and her slow-cooking recipes in chapter 9. Diane's quick dinner recipes are in chapter 8.

Remember, never let more than four or five hours go by without eating a Zone meal or snack. Eat even if you're not hungry. It's also very important to keep a food diary to record winning meals and note other meals that don't go the distance.

LEVEL TWO: Now follow the recipes or different food combinations offered in chapters 3 through 5 to see what it feels like to be in the center of the Zone. It's a good idea to take this step on a weekend, giving you time to get organized, fully stock your kitchen (see chapter 2), and plan your menus. After a week or so, cooking in the Zone will be second nature. Just remember to eat the foods you enjoy. Choose from soups, stir-fries, and stews that you can eat for dinner and have leftovers for lunch the next day. If you prefer to make your dinner in the morning or the night before, this book will tempt you through an entire chapter of slow-cooker recipes. There's even a Can-Do Zone chapter that shows you how to open a can of this and a frozen package of that to put together a quick Zone meal. Read the charts in chapters 3 through 5 to help you put together recipes with simple ingredients.

Most of Rachel's recipes serve about four people, and most of Diane's recipes serve two people. At this point, don't be obsessive about figuring out exactly how much to eat. Just remember the hand-eye method of Zoning, described on page 10.

LEVEL THREE: Once you get comfortable using the recipes and tips in this book, you may want to go on to learn the Zone Food Block method to help you create Zone meals and snacks using all your favorite foods. (A Food Block list begins on page 365.) We list all the good proteins, carbohydrates, and fats that keep you in the Zone due to their low glycemic load. In other words, they don't cause an insulin spike that leaves you light-headed, hungry, lethargic, and in carbo hell. The glycemic load is an excellent guide to how much insulin you will generate in a given meal. Consider 1 cup of brown rice, 1 medium apple, and 1 cup of cooked broccoli. All three choices seem pretty healthy, but don't be fooled. The impact on insulin from each is dramatically different. The glycemic load is shown in the chart on the following page. Note that the 1 cup cooked brown rice will have the same effect on insulin as six sugar cubes.

If you want to be more precise, you need to know how much of a certain macronutrient (protein, carbohydrate, or fat) is needed for a typical woman and a typical man. Most women use the formula of 3–3–3. That means three protein blocks, three carbohydrate blocks, and three monounsaturated fat blocks in every Zone meal. If the use of the word *block* confuses you, think of *selections* instead. Each selection in

CARBOHYDRATE	GLYCEMIC LOAD	SUGAR CUBE UNITS
1 cup broccoli	1.5	0.6
1 sugar cube	2.4	1
1 medium apple	9.7	4
1 cup cooked pasta	30	12.5
1 medium potato	50	21
1 cup whole grain rice	56	23
1 large bagel	70	29

the Food Block Guide is one block. For example, one ounce of chicken equals one block, which means that a woman would serve herself three ounces of chicken. That's three protein blocks. Then she would choose three blocks of carbohydrates and three blocks of heart-healthy monounsaturated fat, which include olive oil, almonds, and avocado. Snacks contain one block each of protein, carbohydrate, and fat.

For men, the formula is usually 4–4–4. That means the typical man will eat four blocks (selections) of protein, four blocks of carbohydrates, and four blocks of fat at every meal, and one block of each for snacks.

It helps at this point to explain how much fat you'll eat each day. You won't be consuming vats of fat. One block of olive oil, for example, is only ⅓ teaspoon, and six peanuts equal one block.

To find out exactly how many blocks you need, log onto our website www.drsears.com to make sure you are, indeed, a "typical" man or woman. You'll find a body fat calculator under the Zone Tools category. You may also use the conversion charts on page 380.

No adult should consume fewer than three blocks of protein, carbohydrate, and fat per meal. The chapters on breakfasts, lunches, and dinners give charts that tell you how to put together a Zone meal using the block method. Once you've started to use Zone Food Blocks, you can take more care when filling out your food diary after every meal. If you feel hungry and loopy two or three hours after your last meal, you ate too many carbohydrates. Remove one block of carbohydrate, but keep the protein and fat content the same the next time you eat that exact same meal. If, on the other hand, you feel hungry but alert, you ate too few carbohydrates at your last meal. Add a block of carbohydrate the next time you have that exact same meal. Believe me, keeping a diary is worth the effort. In a matter of weeks you will have an impressive list of meals that you enjoy and that keep you in the Zone.

LEVEL FOUR: Gram it. When you take this final Zone step, new food horizons will open before your eyes. You'll be able to take a can of soup, add some turkey meatballs or soy sausages, and know how much fruit you'll need to add for a quick lunch. You'll be able to find out which breads have the lowest carbohydrate count. Remember, the Zone dietary program doesn't ban bread altogether. You should just eat it in moderation. By using the gram method, you'll be able to get the most cluck for the buck (or slice for the glycemic price). In the Zone Food Block list on page 365, we've done all the gramming for you. By knowing the gram method yourself, you can look at the label on any package or can and know exactly how close that product is to getting you into the Zone.

Here's how to calculate grams in the Zone. One block of protein equals 7 grams, which means a typical woman will eat 21 grams of protein per meal (7 grams × 3 blocks), and a typical man will need 28 grams (7 grams × 4 blocks). One block of carbohydrate equals 9 grams, which means that a woman requires 27 grams per meal (9 × 3), and the typical man needs 36 (9 × 4). When calculating the carbohydrate content, subtract the amount of fiber in the product. For example, the back of a can will give a total carbohydrate count of, say, 42, and a dietary fiber count of say, 8. For Zoning purposes the amount of carbohydrate to be counted is 34.

One fat block equals 3 grams, which means women need 9 grams of fat per meal, and men need 12. Calculating the number of grams in a fat block has always been confusing for Zoners. When using the Zone Food Block Guide, note that fat is given a value of 1.5 grams. That is to give some wiggle room when there is hidden fat in the low-fat protein selection. When using strictly the gram method give fat the value of 3 grams per block.

So here's how to put it all together.

Start with a 19-ounce can of soup, such as Progresso Beef Barley. Now look at the label: 20 grams protein, 20 grams carbohydrate (26 grams total carbohydrate minus 6 grams dietary fiber), and 8 grams fat. Remember, for each meal, a typical woman should eat 21 grams of protein, 27 grams of carbohydrate, and 9 grams of fat. That means the can of soup has about the right amount of protein (round the number up or down) and fat blocks, but one block of carbohydrates is needed. Eat ½ cup of grapes, and it's a Zone meal. Men (28 grams protein, 36 carbs, and 12 fat), however, will have to add more to the meal. Suggestions could include 1 piece of string cheese, 1 cup of grapes, and maybe 6 peanuts. That would bring the meal into the Zone for men. It also shows you how substantial a Zone meal is.

Nutrition Facts

Amount Per Can

Fat	8g
Total Carbohydrate	26g
Dietary Fiber	6g
Protein	20g

Throughout this book, our gramming lesson will continue, allowing you to grab just what you need before you head out the door for work. Go slow. Make sure you understand the various steps you've taken, and you'll quickly bring your knowledge of the Zone to a higher level.

More than 4 million Zone books have been sold since *The Zone* was published in 1995. So how many people are in the Zone? It's hard to tell, even though it's ranked the number-one diet in Hollywood. We hope that the several different degrees of Zoning offered in this book will help many, many more people to become Zoners. Which is the best method? It's up to you. We began the Zone in 1988 by simply eliminating or vastly reducing starch from our meals. We then used the Zone Food Block Guide and realized that the protein we should eat should fill about one-third of our plate, and vegetables and fruit should fill the other two-thirds. We quickly became attuned to the hand-eye method and have been using that for years now. We use the gram method when considering a packaged food or a new food not on the Zone Food Block list. Whatever step you choose to take, you're making a good decision. The more complicated Zone calculations just give you more accurate Zone meals (and thus greater benefits) and more freedom to create Zone meals from a greater variety of foods.

Now it's time to stock your pantry and also stalk your pantry, throwing away foods that are naughty, not nice. Chapter 2 allows you to choose the foods you like to eat. Chapters 3 through 5 give simple calculations for breakfasts, lunches, and dinners in the Zone. You might even want to take a peek at chapter 8, "The Can-Do Zone," for the simplest Zone meals ever.

2

Zoning Your Kitchen

No two cooks are the same; some only want to use the freshest ingredients, while others want to open a can or defrost a frozen entrée. When you begin to Zone your kitchen, look over the lists of Zone-favorable proteins, carbohydrates, and fats in the breakfast, lunch, and dinner chapters of this book and buy the foods that you and your family really like. Also stock up on the types of foods that fit your cooking style, but only what you'll use before it spoils. It's much easier to begin if you have Zone-favorable protein, carbohydrates, and fats at your disposal. Pack away or give away all those tempting foods, such as candy, pasta, potato chips, rice, and the like that are likely to become roadblocks to your quest to enter the Zone. Then you'll be ready to take the fateful first step that occurred in the Sears household in 1988 as the Zone philosophy emerged.

Remember, the key to every Zone meal is to have adequate levels of low-fat protein, about the size and thickness of the palm of your hand. Next come carbohydrates—primarily vegetables and fruit and a moderate amount of selected grains. The best grains allowed in the Zone dietary program are steel-cut oatmeal and barley. Plan to fill about two-thirds of your plate with Zone-favorable carbohydrates. Then add a dash of heart-healthy monounsaturated fat, such as olive oil, nuts, or avocado.

SHOPPING GUIDELINES

One unfortunate shopping practice of which many of us are guilty is buying lots of fresh vegetables and then seeing them spoil before we get around to using them. Here are some shopping, stocking, and storing tips, provided by Rachel Albert-Matesz.

1 Buy eggs and dairy products once every week or two, as needed. Check the "sell-by" date on packages.

2 Shop for fresh fruits and vegetables at least once or twice a week.

3 Frozen vegetables and fruits keep for months in the freezer. The limiting factor is the size of your freezer. If space permits, you may want to stock up so you don't have to shop for these more than once every two to four weeks.

4 Purchase fresh fish, poultry, and meat several times a week. You can freeze fresh meat, poultry, and fish (provided it is tightly wrapped) for later use if the meats have not been previously frozen. Buying and freezing multiple packages is a great time-saver. If you are using Zone Food Blocks, dividing meat into portion sizes saves even more time.

5 Frozen fish, poultry, and meat may be purchased once a week, once a month, or once every few months. Since these items will keep well in the freezer for six to twelve months, you may want to stock up, particularly when your favorite cuts and varieties are on sale.

6 Protein powders will last for many months, so buy them as you need them. Stock up on large canisters if you use protein powders daily; you'll save money.

7 Shop for bottled condiments, canned vegetables, tomato sauce, canned beans, steel-cut oatmeal, barley, and vegetables as often as you like. Since they keep well at room temperature for more than a year (before opening or cooking), you may want to buy the items you use most in duplicate or triplicate, to reduce shopping frequency to once every three to six weeks.

8 If your dried herbs and spices are several years old, you'll do well to toss them into the trash or compost heap and start over. If you buy

quality dried herbs and spices, they should remain flavorful and fragrant for up to a year. Buy more as needed.

9 Buy nuts, seeds, and unrefined oils as often as you like but definitely store them in the refrigerator or freezer to retard spoilage. Olive oil does not have to be refrigerated.

SHOPPING LIST

Protein

Eggs

Whole eggs

Liquid egg whites

Powdered egg whites, plain

Egg white protein powder: plain, vanilla, or chocolate

Storage tips: Eggs refrigerated in the carton generally keep better than eggs stored in the egg compartment of the fridge, where they may absorb odors from other foods. Store dried powdered egg whites and egg white protein at room temperature. Store liquid egg products in the refrigerator or freezer.

Dairy products

Whey protein powder, vanilla or chocolate if desired

Parmesan cheese, low-fat

Mozzarella cheese, low-fat or part-skim

Cheddar cheese, low-fat or part-skim

Monterey Jack cheese, low-fat or part-skim

Swiss cheese, low-fat or part-skim

Feta cheese, low-fat or part-skim

Blue cheese, low-fat or part-skim

Roquefort, low-fat or part-skim

Goat cheese, low-fat or part-skim

Yogurt, plain, low-fat (contains equal amounts of protein and carbohydrate)

Cottage cheese, plain, low-fat

Soy milk, plain, low-fat (Edensoy Original Soy Milk has the best macronutrient profile and flavor)

Soy cheese, low-fat

Storage tips: Refrigerate cheese in its original packaging, or cut blocks of cheese into 1-ounce cubes, or grate or crumble, then weigh, for ease of serving. Store whey protein at room temperature.

Fish (fresh, frozen, and canned)

Cod

Clams

Crabmeat

Haddock

Lobster

Tuna steaks

Salmon, center-cut fillets or steaks

Sardines

Sea bass steaks or fillets

Scallops

Snapper

Shrimp, peeled and deveined

Shrimp, peeled and ready to cook

Salmon burgers, frozen

Tuna burgers, frozen

Tuna, water-packed, salt-free

Storage tips: Refrigerate fresh fish and use within three days or freeze. Use smoked fish within three to five days or freeze. Use frozen fish within five months; thaw frozen fish in bowls, loaf pans, or baking dishes with sides. Cook within three days; do not refreeze.

Poultry (fresh or frozen)

Ground chicken and turkey, skinless, preferably breast meat

Ground ostrich

Turkey breast, whole, boneless or bone in

Chicken breast: halves, fillets, and boneless skinless breasts

Chicken thighs, boneless or bone-in

Cornish game hens

Sausage, low-fat links: turkey, chicken

Meat

Ground beef, 7 percent or less fat

Ground bison/buffalo

Beef or buffalo steaks (round or loin cuts)

Stew meat: beef, buffalo, ostrich

Pork loin, roast, steaks, or cutlets

Pork chops, boneless or bone in

Sausage, low-fat links: buffalo

Storage tips: Refrigerate fresh meat and poultry or thaw, if frozen, in bowls, loaf pans, or baking dishes with sides. Cook fresh or thawed meat within three days. Consume cooked meats within four days or freeze. Use frozen meat within six months.

Meat and poultry (ready to eat)

Deli-style turkey breast

Roast beef

Rotisserie chicken

Roast turkey

Storage tips: Refrigerate in closed containers and use within one week or follow package instructions.

Meat alternatives

Vegetarian sausage links

Vegetarian-style "crumbles"

Vegetarian ham, roast beef, or turkey-style slices

Carbohydrates

Vegetables (frozen)

Broccoli

Cauliflower

Broccoli/cauliflower blend

Midwestern blend (broccoli, cauliflower, carrot)

Stir-fry blend

Italian blend

California blend

Brussels sprouts

Spinach, cut leaf

Hardy greens: kale, collards, mustard, turnip greens

Onions, chopped white

Onions, pearl, whole

Carrots, sliced

Bell peppers, sliced

Artichoke hearts

Winter squash puree

Peas*

Corn*

Potatoes*, french fry cut

*Note: These high-glycemic vegetables are used in very small amounts in several recipes, not as the primary vegetable, but as flavoring.

Vegetables (fresh)

Lettuces: romaine heads or hearts, red leaf, green leaf, oak leaf, Bibb, and Boston

Salad greens: radicchio, endive, escarole, arugula

Spinach, baby or flat-leaf

Salad green mixes: Mesclun, spring, baby greens, and Italian

Asparagus

Broccoli, bunches or precut florets

Cauliflower, heads or precut florets

Cabbage, red or green heads, or shredded

Coleslaw mix

Precut stir-fry vegetables

Onions: red, yellow, and white

Shallots

Mushrooms: button, cremini, or shiitake, whole or precut

Celery, bunches, hearts, or precut sticks

Carrots, regular, precut sticks, and shredded*

Baby carrots*

Jicama

Turnips, regular or baby

Cucumbers, regular or English/burpless

Tomatoes, cherry, plum, Roma, beefsteak

Scallions (green onions)

Bell peppers, red, yellow, orange, and green

Zucchini or summer squash

Eggplant

Potatoes*

Corn on the cob*

*Note: These high-glycemic vegetables are used in very small amounts in several recipes, not as the primary vegetable, but as flavoring.

Vegetables (dried)

Sun-dried tomato halves, bottled in olive oil or dry pack

Sun-dried tomato bits, dry pack

Dried onion flakes

Dried celery bits/flakes

Dried bell pepper bits

Dried parsley

Dried chives

Storage tips: Store dried vegetables in jars and use within three years for best results.

Vegetables (canned or bottled, unsweetened, oil-free)

Tomato paste

Tomatoes, whole, peeled, diced, or pureed

Tomato sauce and pasta sauce

Salsa, mild or spicy

Ketchup, fruit-sweetened

Mushrooms, sliced

Artichoke hearts

Roasted bell peppers or hot peppers

Storage tips: Store bottled products at room temperature. Once opened, refrigerate and use within one to two weeks.

Grains

Whole oat groats

Steel-cut oats

Rolled oats, thick or old-fashioned

Pearl barley

Oat flour

Whole wheat pita pockets, regular or mini-size (store in the refrigerator)

French Meadow Bread (store in the refrigerator or freezer)

Storage tips: Store grains in jars at room temperature or in the refrigerator or freezer. Once cooked, refrigerate and use within five days or freeze to prolong shelflife.

Beans (canned, no-salt, unsweetened)

Chickpeas (garbanzo beans)

Black beans

Small red beans or azuki beans

Kidney beans

Pinto beans

Navy beans

Cannellini or white beans

Lentils

Mixed chili beans

Storage tips: Store cans at room temperature. Once opened, drain, refrigerate in a covered container, and use within four days.

Fruits (frozen, unsweetened)

Berries, blueberries, strawberries, raspberries, or berry blend

Cherries, pitted sweet

Peaches, sliced

Grape, peach, cherry mix

Pineapple cubes

Storage tips: Store in the freezer. Use frozen fruits in smoothies without thawing. To thaw for fruit salad, transfer fruit to a jar or bowl, cover, and refrigerate; it should be soft enough to eat in six to ten hours. If you need them more quickly, microwave them on the defrost setting.

Fruit (fresh)

Apples

Pears

Grapes, seedless red or green

Berries, blueberries, strawberries, raspberries

Cherries

Peaches

Nectarines

Plums

Apricots

Pineapple

Kiwi

Lemons

Limes

Grapefruit

Oranges

Tangerines/Tangelos

Clementines

Storage tips: Refrigerate ripe, fragrant, or soft fruits, and all berries. Store hard and unripe fruits (apples, pears, melons, mangoes, peaches, plums, nectarines, oranges, lemons, and so on), at room temperature. Apples, pears, and citrus fruits may be stored at room temperature for up to a week.

To make hard fruits ripen faster: Store unripe fruit with a ripe apple in a closed paper bag at room temperature. Check daily to avoid mold.

Dried Fruits (sulfite-free, unsweetened)

Raisins*

Dried apricots, whole or halves*

Prunes, pitted*

Dates, pitted*

Note: These high-glycemic products are to be used sparingly as an ingredient in recipes, not as snacks on their own.

Storage tips: Store in jars at room temperature or in the refrigerator.

Fruit juices and jams (bottled)

Lemon juice, bottled

Lime juice, bottled

Apple juice*

Note: This food is not generally recommended in the Zone but is used as a minor ingredient in a few recipes.

Storage tips: Refrigerate bottles after opening.

Healthy nuts, seeds, nut butters (raw or dry roasted, unsalted, unsweetened)

Almonds

Almond butter

Walnuts

Macadamia nuts

Pecans

Cashews

Hazelnuts/filberts

Peanuts

Sesame seeds

Sunflower seeds

Pine nuts

Pine nut butter

Peanut butter

Macadamia nut butter

Cashew butter

Storage tips: Store all nuts in the refrigerator or freezer. Refrigerate nut butters after opening.

To emulsify a new jar of nut butter: Do not pour off the oil on the top of the jar. Transfer contents of jar to a food processor or bowl. Process or stir with a large, sturdy spoon until smooth, then transfer back to the original jar, cover, and refrigerate. Use within one year.

To dry-toast raw nuts: Scatter raw nuts on a dry baking sheet. Toast pine nuts in 325°F oven for 5 to 6 minutes and larger nuts for 10 to 15 minutes, stirring frequently, until aromatic and lightly golden. Allow to cool, then cover and refrigerate. Do not over-toast, or nuts will become bitter and hard to digest.

To dry-toast raw seeds: Stir the seeds constantly in a cast-iron skillet over medium heat until lightly golden and fragrant. Reduce the heat if seeds start to pop out of the pan or burn. Transfer the seeds to a bowl to cool. Refrigerate in jars.

Healthful fats and oils

Extra-virgin olive oil

Refined olive oil (good for cooking)

Toasted sesame oil

Unrefined canola oil

Canola mayonnaise, reduced fat

Nayonnaise (soy-based sandwich spread), regular and/or low-fat

Avocados

Storage tips: Store all oils, except olive, in the refrigerator.

Herbs and spices (fresh)

Ginger root

Garlic

Basil

Parsley

Chives

Dill

Cilantro

Storage tips: Refrigerate fresh herbs, wrapped in moistened, unbleached paper towels or upright in a jar of water. Use within one week. To use, rinse leaves well, remove from stems and mince with a sharp knife or kitchen shears. Or you can wash, spin dry, and mince parsley, chives, and cilantro and store in separate jars in the refrigerator.

Herbs and spices (dried)

Allspice, ground

Nutmeg, ground

Cinnamon, ground

Apple pie spice

Pumpkin pie spice

Bay leaves

Black pepper, ground

Lemon pepper

White pepper, ground

Cayenne, ground

Chipotle, ground (smoked dried jalapeño pepper)

Curry powder

Dry mustard

Coriander, ground

Garlic powder

Dried basil

Dried oregano

Thyme

Tarragon

Marjoram

Sage, rubbed

Rosemary, ground

Chili powder (salt-free)

Ground cumin

Paprika (mild)

Caraway seed

Fennel seeds

Italian herb blend

Herbes de Provence

Poultry seasoning

Onion powder

Pure vanilla extract

Pure maple extract

Poppy seeds

Storage tips: Store dried herbs and spices in jars at room temperature. In order to preserve flavor and freshness, do not store near or on top of a stove, microwave oven, or sunny window.

Sweeteners

Stevia extract powder

Stevia extract liquid

Fructose powder

Storage tips: Store at room temperature.

Condiments and seasonings (bottled)

Capers

Prepared mustards, unsweetened, preservative-free: Dijon, stone-ground, and white (Eden, Westbrae, or Co-op brand preferred)

Spicy mustards: Red Chile-Garlic and Smoked Green Chili White Mustard (True Natural Taste)

Vinegars: red wine, apple cider, balsamic, and brown rice

Umeboshi plum vinegar

Sauerkraut, natural, unsweetened (Eden or Westbrae)

Kosher dill pickles and dill pickle relish, unsweetened, preservative-free (Cascadian Farms)

Ginger juice or grated ginger root, bottled

Hot sauce, mild or spicy

Worcestershire sauce

Horseradish, grated, bottled

Canned or bottled chipotle peppers

Storage tips: Refrigerate after opening.

Miscellaneous staples

Arrowroot starch (a thickener)

Unflavored gelatin

Unsweetened cocoa powder

Liquid hickory smoke seasoning (such as Wright's brand)

Sea salt

Tamari soy sauce

Fantastic Foods Onion Soup & Dip Mix

Fantastic Foods Garlic-Herb Soup & Dip Mix

Annie's Naturals Low-Fat Raspberry Vinaigrette

Annie's Naturals No-Fat Yogurt Dressing

Guar gum or xanthan gum (thickeners)

Baking powder*

Note: Use fresh baking powder. If your baking powder is more than one year old, toss it and buy a new can. When it's old, it won't give a good rise.

Storage tips: Store the products listed above at room temperature.

You may also check out chapter 8, for various frozen and canned ingredients you can store in your pantry or freezer to fix a quick meal when time is tight.

A NOTE ON INGREDIENTS

All of the following products are widely available in natural foods stores and online. Some, such as protein powders, dried and liquid egg white products, and fructose powder and liquid are sold in the health food section of supermarkets or in the baking or dietetic aisle.

Stevia extract powder and liquid

This natural, noncaloric herbal product is extracted from the leaf of a South American plant, *Stevia rebaudiana,* a shrub with incredibly small, sweet leaves that are fifty times sweeter than table sugar. Because the green leaves are slightly bitter, most consumers prefer to use extracts of the stevia leaf, sold as a white powder or clear liquid. These extracts are even more concentrated and one hundred to three hundred times sweeter than sugar.

Because stevia is so concentrated, only minuscule amounts are needed to produce a sweet taste. More is not better. Too much stevia added to a recipe will produce a bitter aftertaste, so it is important to measure meticulously. Although $\frac{1}{16}$ teaspoon might not sound like much (that's half of a $\frac{1}{8}$ teaspoon measure), it's often adequate to sweeten a 12- to 16-ounce fruit smoothie or mug of tea. Similarly, you may only need $\frac{1}{8}$ to $\frac{1}{4}$ teaspoon of stevia extract to sweeten a bowl of oatmeal, and less if you are using a protein powder that is already sweetened. If a range is given in a recipe, always start with the smaller volume, taste, and work your way up if you desire a sweeter taste.

Stevia extract liquids are sold in an alcohol base or a nonalcoholic glycerine base. They may be used interchangeably. Stevia extract powders are sold as pure extracts and in diluted versions, cut with maltodextrin or vegetable or fruit starches, to make them less concentrated and more pourable, for example in individual packets resembling sugar. Different brands may vary in concentration and flavor, depending on how the products were extracted. For this reason, you may need to experiment to find your favorite brand and dosage. If you buy "single serving" packets, don't assume you will need to use the entire packet in a drink or recipe; even these should be added in tiny increments to avoid oversweetening.

Some of the most popular and widely available brands of stevia extract powder and liquid include Wisdom of the Ancients, Kal, Now Foods, Nu Naturals, and Body Ecology. Stevia extract may be stored at room temperature indefinitely, so don't toss it out after a year or two; it keeps well. Single-serving paper packets may clump unless they are sealed in heavy-duty packaging.

Although this sweet herb, native to Paraguay, has a history of safe use since the sixteenth century, it is relatively new to the Western market, where its widespread use would threaten sales of patented artificial sweeteners. For this reason, the FDA has limited labeling and sales of stevia to the "dietary supplement" category and does not currently allow stevia to be added to commercial products other than protein powders (also sold under the supplement category).

Fructose powder and syrup

This highly refined sweetener is extracted from high fructose corn syrup. It has the lowest glycemic index of all caloric, carbohydrate-containing sweeteners. However, like white sugar it has no other nutrients. Thus, it is best used in very small amounts.

Fructose powder and liquid are fairly interchangeable. In general, you'll want to replace liquid sweeteners with fructose syrup and granulated sweeteners with fructose powder. However, when making salad dressings or smoothies, sweetening hot cereal, or making sauces, you can use either liquid or granulated fructose as the sweetener (substituting one for one for sugar or other sweeteners). In the case of Zone muffins, which call for only a small amount of sweetener, you can safely use either the liquid or the dry version, although the liquid one will add more moisture.

Agavé nectar or syrup

A natural liquid sweetener derived from the agavé plant, agavé nectar or syrup contains the same calorie value of sucrose, but because it's 50 percent sweeter, you can get the same sweetness for fewer calories. Its high fructose (90 percent) and low glucose (10 percent) content gives it a low glycemic rating, which means it's absorbed into the bloodstream more slowly than other sweeteners.

Some glycemic index (GI) tables use white bread as the standard; others use pure glucose. Using white bread as the standard (GI = 100), agavé nectar has a GI of 46. For comparison, honey has a GI of 104, sucrose (white sugar) comes in at 92, and fructose (fruit sugar) at 32. This makes agavé nectar Zone-friendly.

Agavé nectar has a long shelflife stored at room temperature and unlike honey it won't crystallize over time, so it is always easy to pour and measure. Light-colored agavé syrup has a flavor far more mild than honey; the dark amber variety is vaguely reminiscent of maple syrup.

This syrup may be used one for one to replace honey or other liquid sweeteners (¾ of a cup of agavé nectar can replace 1 cup of granulated sugar, provided you reduce the liquids in the recipe by ⅓ to ½ cup, although you won't be using sweeteners in that amount on a Zone diet). In salad dressings, yogurt and fruit sauces, smoothies, or freezer pops, where only a small amount of sweetener is called for, agavé may be used interchangeably with fructose powder or table sugar.

Whey protein

Both human mother's milk and cow's milk contain two kinds of protein—casein and whey—in addition to lactose (milk sugar). Whereas whey protein is the predominant protein in human mother's milk, in cow's milk the ratios are reversed. Whey protein is also the least allergenic portion of cow's milk. Because of its similarity to human milk protein, whey protein has the highest biological value of all proteins, meaning it's the most easily digested and absorbed. Whey protein has the most pleasant flavor and texture of all protein powders on the market. For these and other reasons it has become popular as a dietary supplement, particularly for meal replacement drinks and bars. Individuals who are intolerant of milk (unable to digest lactose or casein) can usually consume whey protein without problems, provided they choose a brand that is 99 percent lactose-free (free of milk sugar).

A 1-ounce portion of whey protein typically contains 21 to 25 grams of protein (the amount found in 3 ounces of lean white meat fish, poultry, or 6 egg whites), 0 to 1 gram of fat, and 0 to 5 grams of carbohydrate, depending upon whether it contains lactose (milk sugar), and how it is sweetened. Stevia is ideal (see page 39), because it is free of calories and carbohydrates, but it's not an artificial sweetener. Products sweetened with fructose (see page 40) typically contain between 3 and 5 grams of carbohydrate per 1-ounce portion.

Look for a brand of whey protein with the simplest and fewest ingredients. The best brands are sweetened with the herbal supplement stevia or fructose. If you have trouble digesting lactose (if it causes you gas, bloating, diarrhea, and other unpleasant effects), look for a brand advertised as 99 percent lactose free. Flavored whey protein is generally more readily accepted and more pleasant tasting than unflavored. Choices typically include vanilla, chocolate, and strawberry.

Some of the best-tasting brands sweetened with stevia include Jay Robb Enterprises' hormone-free whey protein and the Wild Oats brand. Other stevia-sweetened brands include Fat Flush Whey Protein and Body Wise. These products cost more than fructose-sweetened products but have a smoother flavor with no aftertaste. A widely available whey protein sweetened with fructose is Optimum Nutrition Natural Whey Protein.

Avoid cheap, off-brand whey protein sold in bulk in markets and natural foods stores; it usually has an awful metallic or chalky taste. Also note that *whey powder* is not the same as *whey protein powder*. Although whey powder comes from milk, it is not high in protein (it's rich in milk sugar, a carbohydrate); it has a very strong flavor, and contains carbohydrates that cause gas and bloating for many individuals, particularly when used in large amounts or by those who are lactose intolerant.

Store whey protein at room temperature, in a cool place, away from the stove, radiators, and other appliances, and use by the expiration date. Serving sizes for protein powders are customarily listed as 1-ounce scoops, rather than as a volume measurement, because different brands vary in weight. You don't need a scale to follow the recipes, since all protein powder canisters come with a 1-ounce scoop. Just remember that 7 grams of protein equal 1 block.

Egg white protein powder

This is the protein powder of choice for those who choose to avoid all dairy products. Because it is made from dried powdered egg whites, it has a high biological value and is easier to digest than protein powders made from soy or other legumes. Egg white protein is fat free. Its relatively high sodium content comes from the naturally occurring sodium found in egg whites.

Egg white protein is sold unflavored and in vanilla and chocolate. Although many brands are sweetened, some companies, such as Jay Robb Enterprises, sell both an unsweetened variety (which you'd want to sweeten with stevia, agavé, or fructose powder, as suggested in the recipes in this book), as well as stevia-sweetened chocolate and vanilla egg white protein powders. As with whey protein, brands with the simplest and fewest ingredients are best. Some companies add bromclain (enzymes from pineapple, papaya, and other fruits) to their protein powders to aid digestion; this is harmless and may in fact be helpful.

A 1-ounce portion of egg white protein typically contains 24 to 25 grams of protein (the amount found in 3 ounces of lean white meat fish, poultry, or 6 egg whites), 0 grams of fat, and 0 to 5 grams of carbohydrate, depending upon whether and how it is sweetened. Stevia is ideal (see page 39) because it is free of calories and carbohydrates, but it's not an artificial sweetener. Products sweetened with fructose (see page 40) typically contain between 3 and 5 grams of carbohydrate per 1-ounce portion.

Store this product in a cool place at room temperature and use by the expiration date. Note that all protein powder canisters come with a 1-ounce scoop, so you don't need a scale to follow the recipes. Serving sizes for protein powders are customarily listed as 1-ounce scoops, rather than as a volume measurement, because different brands vary in weight and volume.

Dried powdered egg whites

This is a fat-free, cholesterol-free protein source you can reconstitute with water and stock or broth and use anywhere you'd normally use fresh eggs: in scrambles, omelets, quiches, casseroles, to bind meatloaf or meatballs, and so on.

Commercial dried powdered egg whites are pasteurized (no longer raw) so you needn't worry about salmonella. Look for a brand that contains no added ingredients, such as Now Foods, Just Whites, or Hickman's, sold in natural foods markets and the health food section of some supermarkets in the baking aisle. Also look for Optimum Nutrition's Egg D'Lite, which is instantized and contains lecithin, so it dissolves more readily in cool or cold liquids.

Although the instructions on packages and canisters may say you can reconstitute this products in cold water, dried powdered whites dissolve more readily in warm liquids, and in a blender or food processor, or a bowl with an immersion blender, unless the product is "instantized."

Because dried powdered egg whites are fat free and dehydrated, they are stable at room temperature, where they may be kept for several years without risk of spoilage.

> 2 teaspoons powdered whites contain 3.2 g protein, 14 calories, 51 mg sodium = 1 egg white

> 1 tablespoon (3 teaspoons) powdered whites contains 6 g protein, 21 calories, 75 mg sodium = 1 medium egg or 2 egg whites

4 teaspoons powdered whites contain 6.4 g protein, 28 calories,
102 mg sodium = 1 egg or 2 egg whites

To replace whole eggs or fresh whites, follow the proportions below

Dried whites	plus water	replaces this amount of eggs
2 teaspoons	2 tablespoons	1 white
4 teaspoons	¼ cup	2 whites or 1 whole egg
2 tablespoons	¼ cup + 2 tablespoons	3 whites
8 teaspoons	½ cup	4 whites or 2 whole eggs
¼ cup	¾ cup	6 whites or 3 whole eggs
⅓ cup	1 cup	8 whites or 4 whole eggs
½ cup	1½ cups	12 whites or 6 whole eggs

Note: Use warm water or juice if whisking dried, powdered egg whites in a bowl. Use cold, cool, or warm liquid if mixing in a blender or food processor. The latter produces the best results.

Liquid egg whites

Like dried powdered egg whites and egg white protein, liquid egg whites are pasteurized, so you don't have to worry about salmonella poisoning. These products are similar to Egg Beaters but contain no added flavorings, colorings, or other additives. Although liquid egg whites are not dairy products, they are sold near the eggs in the dairy cooler and must be refrigerated.

Use these the way you'd use whole eggs or fresh egg whites. Two tablespoons of liquid egg white will replace one egg white. One-quarter cup of liquid egg white can stand in for one whole egg or two egg whites in a recipe.

Some of the most widely available brands include Hickman's, Eggology, and Egg Whites International.

Dried beans

Dried beans are incredibly economical, but they do require advance prep, as shown in the instructions below. It's not as complicated as it sounds, once you cultivate the habit, but it does require planning ahead.

Canned beans are infinitely more convenient than dried. There's no sorting, rinsing, draining, soaking, or cooking required. You just open the can, drain off the liquid, and the beans are good to go. The down side is the cost. It's a tradeoff. Pay less and put more time into the prep, or pay more and skip the prep. Consider the cost/time ratio and decide which one suits your cooking style, schedule, and budget. Even if you do opt for the do-it-yourself approach, you can still benefit from stashing several cans of your favorite beans in the pantry for those days and weeks when you are busy or forget to soak.

When shopping for canned beans, look for products with simple and few ingredients. The ideal: beans and water (kelp or kombu and sea salt are optional). Avoid canned bean products that contain sugar, honey, molasses, and other sweeteners, starches, maltodextrin, and oils, many of which only add excess carbohydrate and/or fat and calories.

Beans are good keepers. Store both canned beans and dried beans at room temperature. Use within several years of purchase. Check canned products for an expiration date.

Although you can cook beans in quantity and freeze them in small containers for use in soups, stews, casseroles, meat loaves, chili, or bean dip, if you plan to use the beans in a salad, you won't want to use frozen beans. The reason? Freezing causes the cell wall to burst, making the beans less attractive, more mushy, watery, and less flavorful. So for salads, you really need to use freshly cooked or canned beans.

PREPARING DRIED BEANS

Prep: 10 minutes
Soaking: 6 to 8 hours or overnight
Cooking: ½ to 1 hour in a pressure cooker; 1 to 3 hours on top of the range
Yield: 2 cups dried beans makes approximately 4 cups cooked

1 Sort the beans to remove small stones, rinse in a bowl of water, and drain. Soak 2 cups of dried beans in 4 cups of cool or cold filtered water for 6 to 8 hours or overnight at room temperature.

2 Drain off the soaking water and rinse the beans again. Add 2 cups fresh water and 1 bay leaf or a 4-inch strip of kelp or kombu sea vegetable. Cover the pot, bring to a boil, reduce the heat, and simmer small beans (navy, aduki/adzuki, or lentils) for 1 hour or large beans (kidney, red, black, white beans, or chickpeas or garbanzo beans) for 2 to 3 hours, or until tender, adding additional water if necessary to keep beans covered. Alternatively, pressure-cook small beans for 30 minutes or large beans for 1 hour.

3 If desired, remove the lid and simmer away the liquid or use the cooking liquid with the beans in the soup, stew, chili, dip, or other recipe. Refrigerate cooked beans and use within 5 days or freeze for future meals.

3

Breakfasts

When I was growing up, the thought of eating one of my mother's soft-boiled eggs for breakfast made me want to sneak out the back door. My mother insisted I had to eat something before I went to school, but she wisely knew it wasn't going to be eggs and oatmeal (both of which I enjoy for breakfast now). My breakfasts back then usually consisted of a bowl of Campbell's Scotch Broth soup and one-half of a grilled cheese sandwich. Although not quite Zoneful, it wasn't that far off and certainly better than the breakfasts most people in this country eat today: cereal, bagels, and muffins. Your days of eating cold cereal (except for Rachel's recipe for Zoned Muesli, found on page 79) or a bagel are over once you've entered the Zone.

When Barry doesn't have a protein powder and berry shake for breakfast, he likes to eat an eight egg-white omelet, 1 cup of oatmeal, and 1 cup of strawberries to get his four blocks of protein and carbohydrate. I, on the other hand, don't want to eat six egg whites to get my three blocks. What I do is use about two egg whites, add 1 ounce of low-fat cheese, and serve three slices of Canadian bacon on the side. That with some oatmeal and berries makes quite a substantial Zone breakfast.

—*Lynn Sears*

When making your meal plan, remember that breakfast can be lunch or dinner or a 1-block Zone snack hoisted to three or four Zone Food Blocks. For example, a snack is ¼ cup low-fat cottage cheese, ⅓ cup unsweetened applesauce, and 3 almonds. For a 3-block meal, raise it to ¾ cup low-fat cottage cheese, 1 cup applesauce, and 9 almonds. For a 4-block meal, raise it to 1 cup of cottage cheese, 1⅓ cups applesauce, and 12 almonds. (For more snack ideas, go to chapter 6 beginning on page 175.) Whatever you choose, remember to eat breakfast within one hour of waking, and never skip it. You've got to get your Zone clock ticking as you begin your day and not let your blood sugar levels get too low, which tells your brain you're hungry, usually for unfavorable carbohydrates.

SIMPLE BREAKFAST IDEAS

Cottage cheese is an excellent source of protein for breakfast.

- Chop up green onions (it only takes a minute) to put on your cottage cheese.

- Applesauce, blueberries, and Mandarin oranges also give cottage cheese some zip, and you can add enough fruit to make your cottage cheese dish your entire breakfast. Add some crumbled nuts on top for your fat content.

Steel-cut oatmeal is an excellent carbohydrate choice for breakfast, but some people balk at the 30 minutes it takes to cook. The McCann's Irish Oatmeal website gives the following tips on how to reduce the cooking times.

- Microwave: Mix ½ cup steel-cut oats with 2 cups of water in an 8-cup bowl (the size of the bowl is important because it must be large enough to allow the oats to bubble up without spilling over). Seal the bowl with plastic wrap and cook at full power for 5 minutes. Stir and cook for another 5 minutes or so; cooking time may have to be adjusted because microwaves vary in size and power.

- Cook ahead: Prepare five days' worth of oatmeal in advance, storing it in an airtight container in the refrigerator. Reheat it in the microwave on high for 2 to 3 minutes.

- Pre-toast: Place the steel-cut oats in a preheated 300°F. oven for approximately 20 minutes. Return the oats to a tightly covered container and store in a cool place. Toasted oats cook in half the time.

Different toppings make oatmeal taste great, especially berries. Put ½ to 1 cup fresh or defrosted frozen raspberries, blueberries, blackberries, or a mixture of berries on top. Cut back your oatmeal by one block.

For a delicious, savory, unusual flavor, cook your oatmeal in chicken or vegetable broth. It makes it taste wonderful.

Fruits you should avoid, especially when first entering the Zone, are melons, bananas, raisins, mangoes, and other tropical fruits, which have a high glycemic level. Defrosted frozen berries work the best for most people. Everybody's biochemistry is different. Some stay in the Zone eating a small wedge of cantaloupe; others do not. That's why keeping a food diary is so important, as we talked about in chapter 1.

All **breads** are not created equal. That's important to know if you simply have got to have a piece of toast occasionally. Read the label to find the carbohydrate gram total, subtract the fiber, and you'll get a true carbohydrate measure. Then make sure that the carbs in the bread don't add up to more than one-third of your breakfast carbohydrates. While a slice from one loaf of bread may add up to two blocks, a slice from a different loaf may add up to only one. We recently found a selection of breads from French Meadow Bakery in Minneapolis; each slice of the bread is as close to the Zone as you're going to find.

Wasa crackers can also give you that taste of bread you want without loading on the carbs. Melt 1 ounce of cheese on top. The bread can count for one-third of your breakfast carbohydrates, but please don't make bread the entire carbohydrate portion of your breakfast. Throw in two blocks of fruit, such as one apple or one orange. A selection of favorable breakfast carbohydrates is included in this chapter.

Nutrition Facts		Nutrition Facts	
Amount Per Slice		Amount Per Slice	
Fat	2g	Fat	1.5g
Total Carbohydrate	11g	Total Carbohydrate	17g
Dietary Fiber	4g	Dietary Fiber	3g
Protein	6g	Protein	4g

French Meadow Women's Bread   **Arnold Natural**
There are other varieties   **100% Whole Wheat White**

It's a good idea to keep your loaf of bread in the freezer. For one thing, if you're in the Zone, your bread will turn green before you use it up if it's not frozen. For another thing, you'll be less tempted to reach for a piece of bread if it's frozen solid.

Now that we've gone through some general breakfast tips, we'll put some breakfasts together, using protein, carbohydrate, and fat blocks. While you familiarize yourself with what is protein and what is carbohydrate, remember our favorite Zone ditty: "Protein moves around, and carbohydrates grow in the ground." A complete Zone Food Block Guide is located on page 365.

Let's choose our protein portion of breakfast first.

Women should choose any combination that gives a total of three blocks of protein

Men should choose any combination that gives a total of four blocks of protein

1 block

¼ cup cottage cheese **or** egg substitute

1 ounce lean Canadian bacon **or** low-fat cheese

2 egg whites **or** soy sausage links

7 grams protein powder

1 soy sausage patty **or** 1 stick string cheese

1½ ounces deli turkey **or** deli ham **or** deli chicken

1 ounce cooked turkey **or** chicken **or** ham

3 strips of turkey bacon

You don't have to follow the breakfast list for breakfast protein. If you want to eat deli turkey or ham or cooked chicken, turkey, or ham left over from last night's dinner, go right ahead.

A typical woman might choose one of the following for her breakfast protein:

- ¾ cup cottage cheese **or**

- 21 grams of protein powder **or**

- ½ cup egg substitute mixed with 1 ounce of low-fat cheese

A typical man might choose:

- ¾ cup cottage cheese and one soy sausage patty **or**

- 28 grams protein powder **or**

- ¾ cup egg substitute with 1 ounce of low-fat cheese

Now choose the carbohydrate portion of your breakfast. Here are some examples.

Women should choose any combination that gives a total of three blocks of carbohydrate

Men should choose any combination that gives a total of four blocks of carbohydrate

1 block

⅓ cup slow-cooking oatmeal **or** unsweetened applesauce **or** fruit cocktail packed in water

¼ cup chickpeas **or** hummus

½ apple **or** orange **or** grapefruit **or** nectarine **or** orange **or** pear

½ cup blueberries **or** boysenberries **or** canned peaches in water

1 kiwi **or** peach **or** plum **or** tangerine

1 cup raspberries **or** strawberries

1 piece of toast (9 grams). Do not have more than one piece of toast for breakfast.

A typical woman might choose one of the following for her breakfast carbohydrate:

- 1 cup unsweetened applesauce **or**

- 1 cup blueberries and 1 piece of toast (9 grams carb) **or**

- ⅔ cup slow-cooking oatmeal with ½ cup blueberries stirred in

A typical man might choose:

- 1⅓ cups unsweetened applesauce **or**

- 1 cup blueberries, 1 piece of toast (9 grams carb), and ½ an orange **or**

- 1 cup slow-cooking oatmeal with ½ cup blueberries stirred in

The final element of a Zone breakfast is adding some fat to the meal.

Women should choose any combination that gives a total of three blocks

Men should choose any combination that gives a total of four blocks

1 block

⅓ teaspoon olive oil

½ teaspoon almond butter **or** natural peanut butter

1 teaspoon slivered almonds **or** natural peanut butter

1 macadamia nut

1 tablespoon avocado **or** guacamole

2 cashews

3 olives **or** pistachios **or** almonds

6 peanuts

The fat portion of the meal for the typical woman might be:

- 3 macadamia nuts **or**

- 1½ teaspoons natural peanut butter **or**

- 1 teaspoon olive oil

The fat portion for a typical man might be:

- 4 macadamia nuts **or**

- 2 teaspoons natural peanut butter **or**

- 1⅓ teaspoons olive oil

Putting It All Together

For breakfast a typical woman might eat one of the following combinations:

- ¾ cup cottage cheese with 1 cup of applesauce and 3 macadamia nuts crushed on top

- 21 grams of protein powder blended with 1 cup blueberries and 1 piece of toast topped with 1½ teaspoons of natural peanut butter
- ½ cup egg substitute sautéed in 1 teaspoon olive oil mixed with 1 ounce of shredded low-fat cheese, ⅔ cup slow-cooking oatmeal with ½ cup blueberries

A breakfast for a typical man might be:

- ¾ cup cottage cheese with 1 cup applesauce mixed in and 3 macadamia nuts crumbled on top, plus 1 soy sausage patty
- 28 grams protein powder blended with 1 cup raspberries and 1 cup blueberries and 1 piece of toast topped by 2 teaspoons natural peanut butter
- ¾ cup egg substitute sautéed in 1⅓ teaspoons olive oil and mixed with 1 ounce of low-fat shredded cheese, 1 cup slow-cooking oatmeal, with ½ cup blueberries

Rachel Albert-Matesz has provided the following wonderful breakfast recipes, including muffin and smoothie recipes that will make breakfast a snap. You'll love her Zoned Muesli.

BREAKFAST RECIPES

SMOOTHIES AND FREEZES

Peaches and "Cream" Sundae

Rachel Albert-Matesz

Prep: 10 minutes   **Yield:**   4 (4-block) meals

Here's a simple way to dress up peaches for breakfast. You can mix up the topping the day or night before you need it. While you're at it, transfer the frozen fruit to a bowl or quart mason jar and thaw overnight in the refrigerator, so you can assemble breakfast within minutes.

Block Size	Ingredients
Vanilla "Cream" Sauce	
4 protein, 4 carbohydrate	2 cups organic low-fat yogurt (2⅔ cup if yogurt does not contain nonfat dry milk)
16 fat	16 macadamia nuts, chopped
12 protein	Four 1-ounce scoops vanilla egg white protein **or** vanilla whey protein (about 1 cup)
	1 teaspoon ground cinnamon **or** ½ teaspoon ground nutmeg
	2 teaspoons pure vanilla extract (nonalcoholic) **or** 1 teaspoon pure vanilla in alcohol
	⅛ to ¼ teaspoon stevia extract powder **or** liquid (optional)

Fruit

9 carbohydrate	6¾ cups thawed, frozen sliced peaches **or** 9 large peaches, halved, pitted, and sliced
3 carbohydrate	24 fresh pitted sweet cherries **or** 1 cup thawed, frozen, unsweetened "sweet" cherries

Instructions

1 In a medium bowl, combine the yogurt, macadamia nuts, protein, cinnamon or nutmeg, and vanilla. Stir and taste. Add stevia if protein powder is unsweetened or a sweeter taste is desired. Cover and chill for several hours or overnight if time permits.

2 Divide the peaches among 4 serving bowls. Top with the vanilla "cream" sauce. Garnish with the cherries and serve immediately.

Variation

Substitute 3 additional peaches for the cherries.

Scrambled Eggs and Herbs with Red Sauce and Berry-Peach Smoothie

Rachel Albert-Matesz

Prep: 10 minutes   **Yield:**   4 (4-block) servings
Cooking: 4 to 6 minutes

Berries, peaches, and yogurt make a delicious morning drink. To round out the meal, try the herb-infused egg scramble below.

Block Size	Ingredients
Berry-Peach Smoothie	
2 protein, 2 carbohydrate	1 cup plain, organic low-fat yogurt (1⅓ cups if yogurt does not contain nonfat dry milk)
4 protein	1⅓ ounces vanilla egg white protein **or** whey protein
4 carbohydrate	2 cups fresh or frozen blueberries
3 carbohydrate	2⅓ cups chopped fresh or frozen peaches (not thawed)
2 carbohydrate	4 teaspoons fructose powder
10 fat	5 teaspoons unsalted, unsweetened almond butter
	1 teaspoon pure vanilla extract
	½ teaspoon ground cinnamon **or** ¼ teaspoon ground nutmeg
	¼ teaspoon stevia extract powder (optional)
Scrambled Eggs	
4 protein	4 small to medium free-range eggs
	2 cups filtered water

6 protein	½ cup dried powdered egg whites
	¾ teaspoon garlic pepper
	½ teaspoon ground turmeric
	½ teaspoon ground black pepper
4 carbohydrate	2 cups tomato sauce
6 fat	2 teaspoons olive oil (not extra-virgin)

Instructions

1 Combine the yogurt, protein, blueberries, peaches, fructose powder, almond butter, vanilla, and cinnamon or nutmeg in a blender. Cover and process until smooth, stopping to scrape down the sides with a spatula. Taste and sweeten with stevia to taste. Pour into 4 glasses and set aside.

2 Crack the eggs into blender. Add the water, egg whites, garlic pepper, turmeric, and black pepper. Cover and blend until smooth, stopping to scrape down the sides with a spatula.

3 Heat tomato sauce in a small saucepan over medium heat.

4 Heat the oil in 12-inch skillet over medium-high heat until the oil shimmers. Do not allow it to smoke. Use regular, not extra-virgin, to avoid smoking. Tilt the skillet to coat it evenly with oil. Pour in the egg mixture all at once and reduce the heat to medium-low. As the eggs begin to set, almost immediately, use a spatula to push the cooked portion aside, letting the uncooked mixture run underneath. Repeat as the eggs start to set. Continue cooking, moving the spatula in a circle, until the eggs are cooked throughout but still glossy and moist, 5 to 6 minutes. Do not allow the eggs to become dry. Finished dish should resemble a quarter or half circle. Cut into 4 portions.

5 Transfer the eggs to 4 serving plates and top with warm tomato sauce. Serve with the fruit smoothies.

Variation

Replace ½ cup powdered egg whites and 2 cups water with 12 egg whites or 1½ cups liquid egg product.

MUFFINS

Zoned Apple Spice Muffins

Rachel Albert-Matesz

Prep: 20 minutes   **Yield:**   4 (4-block) servings
Cooking: 20 to 24 minutes

Oats add a moist texture and more soluble fiber than pastry wheat flour, and they also have a lower glycemic index. For oat flour, grind old-fashioned oats in the blender or buy it in a natural foods store.

Block Size	Ingredients
Dry Ingredients	
8 carbohydrate	1⅓ cups oat flour
12 protein	Four 1-ounce scoops vanilla whey protein (about 1 cup)
	1 tablespoon nonaluminum baking powder
	2½ teaspoons apple or pumpkin pie spice
	1 tablespoon grated orange rind (optional)
Wet Ingredients	
4 protein	4 whole eggs **or** 8 egg whites
4 carbohydrate	1⅓ cups unsweetened applesauce
16 fat	5⅓ teaspoons unrefined canola oil
4 carbohydrate	4½ teaspoons agavé nectar (cactus honey) **or** 2 tablespoons plus 2 teaspoons fructose powder or syrup
	2 teaspoons pure vanilla extract

Instructions

1 Preheat the oven to 350°F. Spray a 12-muffin tin with nonstick cooking spray and set aside.

2 Sift the dry ingredients into a 1½-quart mixing bowl. Stir and set aside.

3 Combine the wet ingredients in a blender. Cover and blend until smooth, stopping to scrape down the sides. Or, whisk the wet ingredients in a large mixing bowl. Add the wet ingredients to the dry ingredients. Stir just until evenly mixed, scraping the bottom of the bowl to incorporate the flour and remove lumps. Do not overmix, or muffins will be tough.

4 Spoon the batter equally into the muffin cups.

5 Bake until firm to the touch and golden on top and around the edges, and a toothpick inserted into the center comes out clean, 20 to 24 minutes. Cool, then run a knife around the edges to release the muffins. Cover and refrigerate. Use the muffins within 1 week, or freeze them.

Note: Muffin liners (unless they are unbleached) don't work well; they'll stick unmercifully, and you'll have to eat the paper.

Variation

Snack-size muffins: Divide the batter among 16 muffin tins, filling any empty tins with 2 to 3 tablespoons of water to keep the pan from warping. Bake for 12 to 15 minutes, or until the muffins are done as tested above. Each muffin will contain 1 protein, 1 carb, and 1 fat block—perfect for snacks.

Zoned Chocolate Cherry Muffins

Rachel Albert-Matesz

Prep: 20 minutes   **Yield:**   4 (4-block) servings
Cooking: 20 to 24 minutes

Cherries add a burst of flavor to these Zone-friendly muffins. They make a delicious breakfast home and on the go. They freeze well so you might want to make a batch for convenience. For oat flour, finely grind old-fashioned oats in a blender or buy it from your local natural foods market.

Block Size	Ingredients
Dry Ingredients	
8 carbohydrate	1⅓ cups oat flour
12 protein	Four 1-ounce scoops chocolate whey protein (about 1 cup)
	2¼ teaspoons pumpkin **or** or apple pie spice
	1 tablespoon nonaluminum baking powder
	1 tablespoon grated orange rind (optional)
Wet Ingredients	
4 protein	4 whole eggs **or** 8 egg whites
16 fat	5⅓ teaspoons unrefined canola oil
4 carbohydrate	8 teaspoons fructose powder **or** syrup **or** agavè nectar
2 carbohydrate	⅔ cup unsweetened applesauce **or** apple juice
2 carbohydrate	1 cup pitted sweet red cherries **or** 1 cup frozen pitted unsweetened "sweet" cherries (not thawed), coarsely chopped

Instructions

1 Preheat the oven to 350°F. Spray a 12-muffin tin with nonstick cooking spray and set aside.

2 Sift the dry ingredients into a 1½-quart mixing bowl. Stir and set aside.

3 Combine the wet ingredients (except the cherries) in a blender. Cover and blend until smooth, stopping to scrape down the sides. Or, whisk the wet ingredients in a large mixing bowl. Add the wet ingredients to the dry ingredients. Stir just until evenly mixed, scraping the bottom of the bowl to incorporate the flour and remove lumps. Do not overmix, or muffins will be tough. Gently fold in the cherries.

4 Spoon the batter equally into the muffin cups.

5 Bake until firm to the touch and golden on top and around the edges, and a tooth-pick inserted into the center comes out clean, 20 to 24 minutes. Cool, then run a knife around the edges to release the muffins. Cover and refrigerate. Use the muffins within 1 week, or freeze them.

Variation

Snack-size muffins: Divide the batter among 16 muffin tins, filling any empty tins with 2 to 3 tablespoons of water to prevent warping. Bake for 12 to 15 minutes, or until the muffins are done as tested above. Each muffin will contain 1 protein, 1 carb, and 1 fat block—perfect for snacks.

Zoned Chocolate Zucchini Spice Muffins

Rachel Albert-Matesz

Prep: 20 minutes
Cooking: 20 to 24 minutes

Yield: 4 (4-block) servings

Chocolate and zucchini might sound like an odd combination, but they actually taste great together. As an added bonus, they contain fiber and antioxidants. Oat flour is rich in soluble fiber, low on the glycemic index, and provides a more moist texture than pastry wheat flour.

Block size	Ingredients
Dry Ingredients	
8 carbohydrate	1⅓ cups oat flour
12 protein	Four 1-ounce scoops chocolate whey protein (about 1 cup)
	1 tablespoon nonaluminum baking powder
	2½ teaspoons apple **or** pumpkin pie spice
	1 tablespoon grated orange rind (optional)
2 carbohydrate	3 cups grated zucchini
Wet Ingredients	
4 protein	2 whole eggs plus 4 egg whites
16 fat	5⅓ teaspoons unrefined canola oil
4 carbohydrate	8 teaspoons fructose powder or syrup
2 carbohydrate	⅔ cup unsweetened applesauce

Instructions

1 Preheat the oven to 350°F. Spray a 12-muffin tin with nonstick cooking spray and set aside.

2 Sift the dry ingredients into a 1½-quart mixing bowl. Stir, top with the zucchini, and set aside.

3 Combine the wet ingredients in a blender. Cover and blend until smooth, stopping to scrape down the sides. Or, whisk the wet ingredients in a large mixing bowl. Add the wet ingredients to the dry ingredients. Stir just until evenly mixed, scraping the bottom of the bowl to incorporate the flour and remove lumps. Do not overmix, or muffins will be tough.

4 Spoon the batter equally into the muffin cups.

5 Bake until firm to the touch and golden on top and around the edges, and a toothpick inserted into the center comes out clean, 20 to 24 minutes. Cool, then run a knife around the edges to release the muffins. Cover and refrigerate. Use the muffins within 1 week, or freeze them.

Note: Muffin liners (unless they're unbleached) don't work well; they'll stick unmercifully and you'll have to eat the paper.

Variation

Snack-size muffins: Divide the batter among 16 muffin tins, adding 2 to 3 tablespoons of water to each empty cup. Bake for 12 to 15 minutes, or until the muffins are done as tested above. Each muffin will contain 1 protein, 1 carb, and 1 fat block—perfect for snacks.

Zoned Blueberry Oat Muffins

Rachel Albert-Matesz

Prep: 20 minutes   **Yield:**   4 (4-block) servings
Cooking: 20 to 24 minutes

You can enjoy blueberry muffins and stay in the Zone with this family-friendly recipe. Grind old-fashioned oats in the blender or shop for oat flour in a natural foods store. By all means, make a double batch if you want to have extras on hand in the freezer.

Block Size	Ingredients
Dry Ingredients	
8 carbohydrate	1⅓ cups oat flour
12 protein	Four 1-ounce scoops vanilla whey protein (about 1 cup)
	2¼ teaspoons pumpkin **or** apple pie spice
	1 tablespoon nonaluminum baking powder
	1 tablespoon grated orange rind (optional)
Wet Ingredients	
4 protein	4 whole eggs **or** 8 egg whites
16 fat	5⅓ teaspoons unrefined canola oil
4 carbohydrate	8 teaspoons fructose powder or syrup
2 carbohydrate	⅔ cup unsweetened apple sauce
2 carbohydrate	1 cup fresh **or** 1⅓ cup frozen blueberries (not thawed)

Instructions

1 Preheat the oven to 350°F. Spray a 12-muffin tin with nonstick cooking spray and set aside.

2 Sift the dry ingredients into a 1½-quart mixing bowl. Stir and set aside.

3 Combine the wet ingredients (except the blueberries) in a blender. Cover and blend until smooth, stopping to scrape down the sides. Or, whisk the wet ingredients in a large mixing bowl. Add the wet ingredients to the dry ingredients. Stir just until evenly mixed, scraping the bottom of the bowl to incorporate the flour and remove lumps. Do not overmix, or muffins will be tough. Gently fold in the blueberries.

4 Spoon the batter equally into the muffin cups.

5 Bake until firm to the touch and golden on top and around the edges, and a toothpick inserted into the center comes out clean, 20 to 24 minutes. Cool, then run a knife around the edges to release the muffins. Cover and refrigerate. Use the muffins within 1 week, or freeze them.

Variation

Snack-size muffins: Divide the batter among 16 muffin tins, filling any empty tins with 2 to 3 tablespoons of water to keep the pan from warping. Bake for 12 to 15 minutes, or until the muffins are done as tested above. Each muffin will contain 1 protein, 1 carb, and 1 fat block—perfect for snacks.

EGGS

Egg, Vegetable, and Cheese Pie Italiano and Fruit Salad with Balsamic Dressing

Rachel Albert-Matesz

Prep: 20 minutes   **Yield:**   4 (4-block) meals
Cooking: 25 to 30 minutes

This do-ahead pie tastes great at room temperature or warmed briefly before serving. Try it for breakfast during the week or on a leisurely Sunday morning.

Block Size	Ingredients
Egg, Vegetable, and Cheese Pie	
2 carbohydrate	2 cups diced, no-salt-added, canned tomatoes with juices
1 carbohydrate	1½ cups diced fresh or thawed frozen onion
3 protein	3 ounces grated, part-skim mozzarella cheese
10 fat	30 olives, rinsed, drained, and chopped
4 protein	4 large eggs
	2 cups filtered water
9 protein	¾ cup dried powdered egg whites
	1 tablespoon herbes de Provence **or** Italian herb blend
	3 garlic cloves, minced **or** 1 teaspoon garlic powder
	½ teaspoon ground turmeric
	½ teaspoon ground black pepper **or** ground chipotle (dried smoked jalapeño)

Fruit Salad

½ carbohydrate	2 tablespoons balsamic vinegar
1½ carbohydrate	1 tablespoon agavé nectar **or** 2½ teaspoons fructose powder
	2 teaspoons minced bottled ginger puree
3 carbohydrate	1 cup fresh pitted or thawed frozen cherries
4 carbohydrate	2 cups fresh or thawed frozen grapes
4 carbohydrate	3 cups fresh or thawed frozen melon balls
6 fat	6 teaspoons raw almonds, chopped

Instructions

1 Preheat the oven to 350°F. Coat a 9 x 9 x 2-inch baking pan with nonstick cooking spray. Scatter ¾ cup of the tomatoes, ½ cup of the onion, all of the grated cheese, and the olives on the bottom of the pan.

2 Add the remaining 1¼ cups tomato and juices, the rest of the onion, the eggs, water, egg white powder, and herbs and spices to a blender or the work bowl of a food processor. Cover and blend until smooth and frothy, stopping to scrape down the sides with spatula to incorporate the powder. Pour the mixture into the baking pan.

3 Bake for 25 to 30 minutes or until puffy, firm to the touch in the center, and lightly golden on top.

4 Cut the pie into 4 slices and serve, or cool, cover, and refrigerate for later.

5 In a large bowl, mix the vinegar, agavé nectar or fructose powder, and ginger. Add the fruit and toss. Cover and refrigerate for 1 hour. Divide into 4 serving bowls, garnish with the almonds, and serve.

Variation

• For a dairy-free pie, replace the grated cheese with 4½ ounces cooked salmon.

• Replace ¾ cup dried powdered egg whites and 2 cups water with 18 egg whites or ¼ cup liquid egg product.

Smoky Salmon and Egg Scramble with Veggies and Blueberry-Orange Salad

Rachel Albert-Matesz

Prep: 10 minutes   **Yield:** 4 (4-block) servings
Cooking: 4 to 6 minutes

Natural liquid hickory smoke seasoning makes salmon taste smoky without sodium nitrate, sugar, or excess sodium. Look for this tasty seasoning on the condiment aisle of super-markets.

Block Size	Ingredients
Fruit Salad	
6 carbohydrate	3 cups blueberries, washed and drained
4 carbohydrate	2 seedless oranges, peeled and sectioned
2 carbohydrate	2 tablespoons raisins
2 carbohydrate	1 cup grapes
½ carbohydrate	2½ tablespoons lime juice
6 fat	18 pecan halves, lightly toasted, crumbled
Vegetables	
1½ carbohydrate	One 16-ounce bag Freshlike frozen California blend (broccoli, cauliflower, carrots)
10 fat	30 black olives, rinsed, drained, and sliced
Salmon and Egg Scramble	
4 protein	4 small to medium free-range eggs
	1½ cups filtered water
6 protein	½ cup dried powdered egg whites
	½ teaspoon ground chipotle (smoked dried jalapeño)

½ teaspoon ground turmeric

½ teaspoon dry mustard

½ teaspoon Wright's liquid hickory
   smoke seasoning

6 fat   2 teaspoons olive oil

6 protein   9 ounces drained canned salmon, flaked

Instructions

1 In a large bowl, toss the blueberries, oranges, raisins, grapes, and lime juice. Divide the fruit salad among 4 bowls and garnish with the pecans. Set aside.

2 In a medium saucepan, bring ½ cup water to boil over medium heat. Add the frozen vegetables, cover, return to boil, and reduce the heat. Simmer 8 to 10 minutes, stirring occasionally. Drain and toss with the olives.

3 Crack the eggs into a blender. Add the water, powdered egg white, chipotle, turmeric, mustard, and liquid smoke seasoning. Cover and blend until smooth, stopping to scrape down the sides with spatula.

4 Heat the oil in a 12- to 13-inch skillet over medium heat. The pan must be hot, or the eggs will stick! Tilt the skillet to completely coat bottom and sides of pan. Pour in the egg mixture. Sprinkle with the salmon and reduce the heat to medium. As the eggs begin to set, almost immediately, use a spatula to push the cooked portion aside, letting the uncooked mixture run underneath. Repeat as the eggs start to set. Continue cooking, moving the spatula in a circle, until the eggs are cooked throughout but still glossy and moist, 5 to 6 minutes.

5 Divide among 4 plates and serve immediately.

Variation

If desired, replace ½ cup powdered egg whites and 1½ cups water with 12 egg whites or 1½ cups liquid egg product.

CEREALS

Apple Pie Spiced Oatmeal

Rachel Albert-Matesz

Prep: 10 minutes   **Cooking:** 40 minutes or overnight
Soaking: Overnight   **Yield:**   4 (4-block) meals

You can simmer this cereal first thing in the morning or let it cook all night, while you sleep, so you can wake up to piping-hot breakfast porridge.

Block Size	Ingredients
12 carbohydrate	2 cups old-fashioned rolled oats **or** 1 cup plus 2 tablespoons steel-cut oats (such as McCann's)
4 carbohydrate	2 small apples, cored and diced
	¾ to 1 teaspoon apple pie spice
	4 cups cold, filtered water (4¼ cups for steel-cut oats)
16 protein	Four 1-ounce scoops vanilla egg white protein **or** vanilla whey protein (about 1 cup)
	3 to 5 drops stevia extract liquid **or** ⅛ teaspoon to ¼ teaspoon stevia extract powder (optional)
16 fat	48 pecan or walnut halves, lightly toasted and crumbled

Instructions for overnight cooking—for steel-cut oats only

1 Before going to bed, combine steel-cut oats, spice, and water in 3½-quart slow cooker. Cover and cook on LOW for 7 to 8 hours.

2 In the morning, turn off the heat and add the apples. Let stand for 10 to 15 minutes; the steam will condense and lift the stuck cereal off the bottom of the cooker for ease of clean up.

3 Stir in the protein powder with a large wooden spoon to dissolve all lumps. If too stiff, stir in warm water a tablespoon at a time. Stir in stevia if a sweeter taste is desired. Stir again and divide among 4 serving bowls. Top with nuts and serve.

Instructions for stovetop cooking—for rolled oats only

1 Combine rolled oats, apple, spice, and water in a 2-quart saucepan. Soak, uncovered, overnight.

2 In the morning, cover and bring to a boil over medium heat, without stirring. If using an electric stove, preheat a second burner on low. When the mixture comes to a boil, reduce the heat to low or transfer it to the preheated burner. Simmer, undisturbed, for 30 minutes, then remove from the heat.

3 Allow the cereal to stand, covered, for 10 to 15 minutes. With a large wooden spoon, stir in the protein powder to dissolve all lumps. If too stiff, stir in warm water a tablespoon at a time. Taste. Stir in stevia if a sweeter taste is desired. Divide among 4 serving bowls. Top with nuts and serve.

Note: Some brands of vanilla egg white protein are unsweetened. Taste before you add the stevia and use a light hand; stevia is one hundred to three hundred times sweeter than sugar.

Variation

Replace the apple pie spice with pumpkin pie spice.

Blueberry-Maple Nut Oatmeal

Rachel Albert-Matesz

Prep: 10 minutes   **Cooking:** 40 minutes or overnight
Soaking: Overnight   **Yield:**   4 (4-block) meals

You can simmer this cereal first thing in the morning or leave it to cook all night while you sleep, so you can wake up to piping hot porridge. In the morning just stir in the flavorings and protein powder and top it off with blueberries and nuts.

Block Size	Ingredients
12 carbohydrate	2 cups old-fashioned rolled oats **or** 1 cup plus 2 tablespoons steel-cut oats (such as McCann's)
	¾ teaspoon ground cinnamon
	4 cups cold, filtered water (4¼ cups for steel-cut oats)
16 protein	Four 1-ounce scoops vanilla egg white protein **or** whey protein (about 1 cup)
	2 teaspoons pure maple extract, preferably nonalcoholic
	3 to 6 drops stevia extract liquid **or** ⅛ to ¼ teaspoon stevia extract powder (optional)
4 carbohydrate	2 cups blueberries
16 fat	48 pecan or walnut halves, lightly toasted and crumbled

Instructions for overnight cooking—for steel-cut oats only

1 Before going to bed, combine the steel-cut oats, spice, and water in 3½-quart slow cooker. Cover and cook on LOW for 7 to 8 hours.

2 In the morning, turn off the heat. Let stand for 10 to 15 minutes; the steam will condense and lift the stuck cereal off the bottom of the cooker for ease of clean-up.

3 Add protein powder and maple extract. Stir with a large wooden spoon to dissolve all lumps. If too stiff, stir in warm water, a tablespoon at a time. Taste and add stevia if a sweeter taste is desired. Stir well then divide among 4 serving bowls. Top with berries and nuts and serve.

Instructions for stovetop cooking—for rolled oats only

1 Combine the rolled oats, spice, and water in 2-quart saucepan. Soak, uncovered, overnight.

2 In the morning, cover and bring to a boil over medium heat, without stirring. If using an electric stove, preheat a second burner on low. When the mixture comes to a boil, reduce the heat to low or transfer it to the preheated burner. Simmer, undisturbed, for 30 minutes, then remove from the heat.

3 Allow the cereal to stand, covered, for 10 to 15 minutes. With a large wooden spoon, stir in the protein powder to dissolve all lumps. If too stiff, stir in warm water a tablespoon at a time. Taste. Stir in the maple extract and, if desired, the stevia. Divide among 4 serving bowls. Top with berries and nuts and serve.

Note: Some brands of vanilla egg white protein are sold unsweetened. If you use one of these you will need to add stevia to sweeten. Start with the smallest amount then adjust if needed.

Banana-Nut Oatmeal

Prep: 10 minutes   **Cooking:** 40 minutes or overnight
Soaking: Overnight   **Yield:**   4 (4-block) meals

For convenience, start your cereal cooking before you go to bed. Let it cook all night on low. In the morning, just add protein powder, fruit, and a Zone-friendly fat source and breakfast is ready! If you're heading to the gym, stow your cereal in a thermos so you can dine after your workout.

Block size	Ingredients
12 carbohydrate	2 cups old-fashioned rolled oats **or** 1 cup plus 2 tablespoons steel-cut oats (such as McCann's)
	¾ to 1 teaspoon ground cinnamon **or** apple pie spice
	4 cups cold filtered water (4¼ cups for steel-cut oats)
16 protein	Four 1-ounce scoops vanilla egg white protein **or** whey protein (about 1 cup)
	2 teaspoons pure maple extract, preferably nonalcoholic
	3 to 4 drops stevia extract powder (optional)
4 carbohydrate	1⅓ medium bananas, peeled and sliced
16 fat	48 almond or walnut halves, lightly toasted and crumbled

Instructions for overnight cooking—for steel-cut oats only

1 Before going to bed, combine the steel-cut oats, spice, and water in a 3½-quart slow cooker. Cover and cook on LOW 7 to 8 hours.

2 In the morning, turn off the heat. Let stand for 10 to 15 minutes (the steam will condense and lift the cereal off bottom of the cooker, making it easier to clean up).

3 Add the protein powder and maple extract. Stir with a large wooden spoon to dissolve all the lumps. If the oatmeal is too stiff, stir in warm water a tablespoon at a time. Taste and add stevia if a sweeter taste is desired. Stir well and divide among 4 serving bowls. Top with bananas and nuts and serve.

Instructions for stovetop cooking—for rolled oats only

1 Combine rolled oats, spice, and water in a 2-quart saucepan. Soak overnight, uncovered.

2 In the morning, cover and bring to a boil over medium heat without stirring. If using an electric stove, preheat a second burner on low. When the oatmeal comes to a boil, reduce the heat to low or transfer it to the preheated burner. Simmer, undisturbed, for 30 minutes and remove from the heat.

3 Allow the cereal to stand, covered, for 10 to 15 minutes. With a large wooden spoon, stir in the protein powder and maple extract to dissolve all lumps. If the oatmeal is too stiff, stir in warm water a tablespoon at a time. Taste. Stir in stevia if a sweeter taste is desired. Divide among 4 serving bowls, top with bananas and nuts and serve.

Note: Some brands of vanilla egg white protein are sold unsweetened. If you use one of these you will need to add stevia to sweeten. Start with the smallest amount then adjust if needed.

Zoned Muesli

Rachel Albert-Matesz

Prep: 15 minutes
Soaking: Overnight

Yield: 4 (4-block) meals

Muesli is a cross between hot and cold cereal. Traditionally the oats are soaked overnight in yogurt or kefir (a runnier version of yogurt). In the morning, grated or thinly sliced fresh fruit is added to the soft cereal. The classic Swiss version does not contain protein powder.

Block Size	Ingredients
Oat, fruit, and nut mixture	
7 carbohydrate	1 cup plus 2½ tablespoons old-fashioned, thick rolled oats
4 fat	12 almonds, coarsely chopped
4 fat	12 pecan halves, coarsely chopped
4 fat	12 walnut halves, coarsely chopped
4 fat	4 macadamia nuts, coarsely chopped
2 carbohydrate	2 tablespoons raisins
1 carbohydrate	3 sulfite-free whole dried apricots **or** 6 dried apricot halves, minced
	1 teaspoon apple pie spice **or** ground cinnamon
12 protein	Four 1-ounce scoops vanilla whey protein (about 1 cup)
4 protein, 2 carbohydrate	2 cups plain, low-fat kefir **or** yogurt, preferably organic

Fresh Fruit

2 carbohydrate	1 small apple, cored and grated
2 carbohydrate	1 small pear, cored and grated **or** ⅔ of a ripe banana, sliced
	⅛ to ¼ teaspoon stevia extract powder **or** 3 to 6 drops stevia extract liquid (optional)

Instructions

1 In a dry skillet over medium-low heat, toast the oats and nut pieces until lightly golden and aromatic, stirring all the while, 3 to 5 minutes. In a medium bowl, toss the oats, nuts, raisins, apricots, spice, and protein powder.

2 Before going to bed, add the kefir or yogurt to the oat mixture. Stir, cover, and refrigerate overnight.

3 In the morning, prepare the apple and pear or banana. Stir into the muesli and let stand for 15 minutes. If desired, add a little water. If you prefer a sweeter taste, stir in stevia. Divide among 4 cereal bowls and serve.

FRUIT

Faux Frittata with Fruit Salad

Rachel Albert-Matesz

Prep: 15 minutes   **Yield:**   4 (4-block) meals
Cooking: 10 to 15 minutes

Unlike traditional frittatas, this one is low in fat and calories, and you can cook it completely on top of the stove. Stock up on dried powdered egg whites and dried onion flakes for convenience.

Block Size	Ingredients
Frittata	
4 protein	4 small to medium free-range eggs
	1½ cups filtered water
9 protein	¾ cup dried powdered egg whites
2 carbohydrate	4 plum (Roma) tomatoes **or** 2 large tomatoes, cored and halved
4 carbohydrate	¼ cup dried onion flakes
	½ teaspoon ground turmeric
	½ teaspoon ground chipotle (smoked dried jalapeño) **or** black pepper
	1 teaspoon ground cumin **or** dry mustard
6 fat	2 teaspoons olive oil (not extra-virgin)
3 protein	3 ounces shredded low-fat cheese, such as cheddar or Monterey Jack

Fruit Salad

2 carbohydrate	2 tangerines, peeled and sectioned
4 carbohydrate	2 cups red grapes, halved
4 carbohydrate	3 cups fresh or thawed frozen melon balls
10 fat	10 macadamia nuts, chopped

Instructions

1 Crack the eggs into a blender. Add the water, egg white powder, tomatoes, onion, turmeric, chipotle or black pepper, and cumin or mustard. Cover and blend until smooth and frothy, stopping to scrape down the sides with spatula.

2 In a heavy 12-inch skillet, heat the oil over medium heat until hot but not smoking. Tilt the skillet to coat evenly with oil. If you're cooking with olive oil, make sure it's not extra-virgin, as it smokes too easily.

3 Pour the egg mixture into the skillet, cover, and reduce the heat to medium-low. Cook undisturbed for 12 to 14 minutes, or until slightly puffy and firm on top. Sprinkle with the cheese and remove from the heat. Let rest, covered, for 5 minutes, so that steam condenses in the pan for ease of removal.

4 Meanwhile, in a large bowl, toss together all the fruit salad ingredients.

5 Cut the frittata into 8 wedges and serve with the fruit salad on the side. Cover and refrigerate any leftovers and use within 3 days.

Variation

Replace ¾ cup powdered egg whites and 1½ cups water with 18 egg whites or 2¼ cups liquid egg product.

Fruit Salad with Lemon-Poppy Seed Dressing

Rachel Albert-Matesz

Prep: 15 minutes plus defrost overnight   **Yield:**   4 (4-block) meals

To simplify breakfast, pour the frozen fruit into a large bowl the evening before you need it. Mix in the yogurt sauce and chill overnight. In the morning, all you'll have to do is divvy up the contents.

Block Size	Ingredients
12 carbohydrate	Three 16-ounce bags mixed frozen fruit (peaches, cantaloupe, honeydew melon, red seedless grapes)
4 protein, 2 carbohydrate	2⅔ cups Stonyfield Farm or Horizon plain, organic, low-fat yogurt **or** 2 cups yogurt made with nonfat dry milk solids
12 protein	Four 1-ounce scoops vanilla whey protein (about 1 cup)
	1 rounded tablespoon poppy seeds
	2 teaspoons pure vanilla extract (nonalcoholic)
	½ teaspoon grated lemon rind (yellow part only)
	2 teaspoons fresh lemon juice
	⅛ to ¼ teaspoon stevia extract powder (optional)
2 carbohydrate	1 cup fresh blueberries, rinsed and drained
16 fat	⅓ cup hazelnuts, chopped and lightly toasted, **or** pecans, chopped

Instructions

1 Pour the frozen fruit into a large bowl, cover, and defrost all day or overnight in the refrigerator.

2 In a medium nonmetallic mixing bowl with a lid, combine the yogurt, protein powder, poppy seeds, vanilla, lemon rind, and lemon juice. Stir, taste, and add stevia if a sweeter taste is desired. Cover and refrigerate for several hours or overnight.

3 Stir the fruit, add the blueberries, and divide it among 4 serving bowls. Divide the dressing into 4 portions and spoon it over the fruit. Sprinkle with nuts and serve.

Variation

Substitute 2 sliced fresh peaches, 2 cups cubed fresh honeydew melon, 2 cups cubed fresh cantaloupe, and 2 cups seedless red grapes for the frozen fruit.

Slow-Poached Pears with Vanilla Yogurt Sauce

Rachel Albert-Matesz

Prep: 15 minutes   **Yield:**   4 (4-block) meals
Cooking: 3 hours

To simplify breakfast, cook the pears the day or evening before you need them. Mix up the yogurt sauce and chill overnight. In the morning, assembling breakfast will be effortless.

Block Size	Ingredients
Pears	
8 carbohydrate	4 small ripe (but not mushy) pears
3 carbohydrate	3 tablespoons raisins
1 carbohydrate	3 sulfite-free whole dried apricots **or** 6 dried apricot halves, finely chopped
	⅛ cup filtered water
2 carbohydrates	2 teaspoons fructose powder
	1 teaspoon grated lemon or orange rind **or** ⅛ teaspoon dried lemon or orange rind
	1½ tablespoons finely grated fresh ginger root **or** Hawaii Naturals bottled ginger puree
	1 cinnamon stick
Yogurt Topping	
4 protein, 2 carbohydrate	2⅔ cups Stonyfield Farm or Horizon plain, organic, low-fat yogurt **or** 2 cups yogurt made with added milk solids
12 protein	Four 1-ounce scoops vanilla whey protein (about 1 cup)
	⅛ to ¼ teaspoon stevia extract powder (optional)
16 fat	16 macadamia nuts, chopped

Instructions

1 Using an apple corer, remove the core from the bottom of the pears, leaving the stem intact. Peel the pears and arrange them in a 2½- to 3½-quart slow cooker. Sprinkle with raisins and dried apricots.

2 In a medium bowl, combine the water, fructose, lemon or orange rind, and ginger. Pour the mixture over the pears. Place the cinnamon stick in the middle of the cooker. Cover and cook on LOW for 2½ to 3 hours, or until fork-tender.

3 In a medium bowl, combine the yogurt and protein powder. Stir, taste, and add stevia if a sweeter taste is desired.

4 Transfer the pears to 4 serving bowls. Evenly distribute the cooking juices and dried fruits among 4 serving bowls. Spoon yogurt over pears and garnish with nuts.

Variation

Substitute small baking apples for the pears.

Spinach-Egg Pie with Fruit Salad

Rachel Albert-Matesz

Prep: 20 minutes   **Cooking:** 25 to 30 minutes
Soaking: 3 hours to overnight   **Yield:**   4 (4-block) meals

Here's a great Zone-friendly alternative to quiche. You can make it on a Sunday or an evening during the week and serve it two mornings in a row.

Block Size	Ingredients
Spinach Pie	
1 carbohydrate	8 to 12 sun-dried tomato halves, cut into bite-size pieces with kitchen shears **or** 8 to 12 teaspoons sun-dried tomato bits
16 fat	5⅓ teaspoons extra-virgin olive oil
½ carbohydrate	2½ tablespoons lemon juice
1 carbohydrate	One 16-ounce package frozen spinach, thawed
3 protein	3 ounces grated, part-skim mozzarella cheese (¾ cup)
4 protein	4 large eggs
	2 cups filtered water
9 protein	¾ cup dried powdered egg whites
4 carbohydrate	4 tablespoons dried onion flakes
½ carbohydrate	1 tablespoon dried bell pepper flakes
	1 tablespoon Italian herb blend
	4 garlic cloves, minced **or** 1⅛ teaspoon garlic powder
	½ teaspoon ground turmeric
	½ teaspoon ground black pepper **or** ground chipotle (smoked dried jalapeño)

Fruit Salad

3 carbohydrate	1½ cups cubed fresh or thawed frozen pineapple
3 carbohydrate	1 cup cubed fresh or thawed frozen mango
3 carbohydrate	3 cups fresh or thawed frozen strawberries

Instructions

1 In a small jar, combine the tomatoes, olive oil, and lemon juice. Soak for at least 3 hours at room temperature to soften, or cover and refrigerate overnight.

2 Preheat the oven to 350°F. Coat a 9 x 9 x 2-inch baking pan with nonstick cooking spray. Spread the spinach over the bottom of the pan and sprinkle with the cheese.

3 In a blender or the work bowl of a food processor, combine the eggs, water, egg white, onion flakes, bell pepper flakes, Italian herb blend, garlic or garlic powder, turmeric, and black pepper or chipotle. Cover and blend until smooth, stopping to scrape down the sides with spatula. Stir in the sun-dried tomatoes and liquid. Pour the mixture over the spinach and cheese.

4 Bake for 25 to 30 minutes, or until the center of the pie is firm to the touch, the top of the pie is golden, and a toothpick inserted into the center comes out clean. Serve immediately or cover and chill for later. Cut into 16 slices; 4 slices equal 4 protein blocks.

5 In a large bowl, toss the fruit. Divide among 4 bowls and serve with the spinach pie.

Variation

- Dairy-free pie: Replace the grated cheese with 4½ ounces cooked, drained baby shrimp or salmon.

- Replace ¾ cup dried powdered egg whites and 2 cups water with 18 egg whites or 2¼ cups liquid egg product.

Fruit Salad with Maple Yogurt Sauce

Rachel Albert-Matesz

Prep: 10 minutes   **Yield:**   4 (4-block) meals

Vanilla whey protein powder produces the best results in this recipe. If possible, find a brand such as Jay Robb's All-Natural Vanilla Whey Protein, sweetened with stevia extract powder rather than an artificial sweetener or fructose. The taste will be smoother and you'll avoid the additives. If you use unsweetened protein powder, you may need to add additional stevia.

Block Size	Ingredients
Maple Yogurt Sauce	
4 protein, 4 carbohydrate	2 cups organic low-fat yogurt (⅔ cup if yogurt does not contain nonfat dry milk)
12 protein	Four 1-ounce scoops vanilla egg white protein **or** vanilla whey protein (about 1 cup)
	1 teaspoon pure maple extract (nonalcoholic) **or** ½ teaspoon maple extract in alcohol
	½ teaspoon ground cinnamon **or** ¼ teaspoon ground nutmeg
	⅛ to ¼ teaspoon stevia extract powder or liquid (optional)
Fruit Salad	
3 carbohydrate	3 cups sliced fresh **or** thawed frozen strawberries
3 carbohydrate	3 peaches, halved, pitted, and diced **or** 2¼ cups thawed frozen sliced, unsweetened peaches

3 carbohydrate	1½ cups seedless red or green grapes, halved
	½ teaspoon apple pie spice
3 carbohydrate	1 cup pitted fresh sweet cherries **or** 1 cup thawed frozen, pitted unsweetened "sweet cherries"
16 fat	⅓ cup chopped, lightly toasted pecans

Instructions

1 In a medium bowl, combine the yogurt, protein powder, maple extract, and cinnamon or nutmeg. Stir, taste, and stir in stevia if protein powder is unsweetened and a sweeter taste is desired. Cover and chill for several hours, or overnight if time permits.

2 In a large bowl, combine the strawberries, peaches, grapes, apple pie spice, and cherries. Stir and divide among 4 serving bowls. Top with the maple yogurt mixture. Garnish with the nuts and serve immediately.

Variation

Substitute blueberries for the grapes.

4

Lunches

Although Barry sometimes likes to have a big plate of steamed vegetables with his lunch, that's more of a dinnertime accompaniment to me. Besides, who wants to chop vegetables in the middle of the day? Get real.

—Lynn Sears

Lunch can be the easiest or hardest meal of the day. At home it's a snap. At work, it's a challenge to say the least.

A complete Zone Food Block Guide is located on page 365, indicating countless combinations to use to make Zone meals. Here are a few choices to get you started.

Finding a protein choice for lunch is easy. Just follow the chart below:

Women should choose any combination that gives a total of three blocks or selections.

Men should choose any combination that gives a total of four.

1 ounce skinless chicken **or** turkey breast, **or** game, **or** lean beef

1½ ounces fish (including haddock, bass, cod, salmon, shrimp, scallops, or swordfish)

1 ounce canned tuna packed in water **or** tuna steak **or** sardines

¼ cup low-fat cottage cheese (chopped green onions make it taste much better)

1 ounce low-fat cheese **or** 1 piece low-fat string cheese

1½ ounces ground turkey **or** buffalo **or** beef (less than 10 percent fat)

1½ ounces deli turkey **or** chicken **or** ham

2 ounces firm tofu

3 ounces lean Canadian bacon

Soy products, including burgers, hot dogs, and sausages. Check the label. Each protein block equals 7 grams. Also, take the carbohydrate content into account.

So all you have to do is make three (for women) or four (for men) selections from the protein list. For example, a woman can choose to eat:

- 3 ounces skinless chicken breast **or**
- 3 ounces deli meat and 1 piece of string cheese **or**
- ¾ cup of low-fat cottage cheese

A man might select:

- 4 ounces skinless chicken breast **or**
- 4½ ounces deli meat and 1 piece of string cheese **or**
- 1 cup of low-fat cottage cheese

While it might appear that it's harder to make quick carbohydrate selections, the chart below will make such choices easy.

Women should choose any combination that gives a total of three blocks or selections.

Men should choose any combination that gives a total of four.

¼ cup kidney beans **or** chickpeas **or** black beans **or** hummus

⅓ cup water chestnuts

½ cup salsa **or** tomato sauce

1½ cups chopped onions **or** spaghetti squash

⅓ cup unsweetened applesauce **or** light fruit cocktail **or** Mandarin
    oranges in water

½ apple or grapefruit **or** nectarine **or** orange **or** pear

½ cup blueberries **or** boysenberries **or** grapes **or** peaches canned in
    water

1 kiwi **or** peach **or** plum **or** tangerine

1 cup raspberries **or** strawberries

9 grams of the **bad stuff** (unfavorable carbohydrates) such as bread
    (Check the label and limit these to one block per meal. At best
    you should eat none.)

This means that a woman might choose:

- ¼ cup chickpeas on a small side salad and an apple **or**

- 1 cup blueberries and 1 slice of bread (about 9 grams) **or**

- A fruit salad of 1 cup grapes and ⅓ cup Mandarin oranges

A man might choose:

- ½ cup of chickpeas on a small side salad and an apple **or**

- 1 cup blueberries mixed with 1 sliced peach and one slice of bread **or**

- A fruit salad of 1 cup grapes and ⅔ cups Mandarin oranges

The final component of a Zone meal is the fat.

**Women should choose any combination that gives a total of three
blocks or selections.**

Men should choose any combination that gives a total of four.

⅓ teaspoon olive oil

½ teaspoon tahini **or** almond butter **or** natural peanut butter

1 teaspoon slivered almonds

1 macadamia nut

1 tablespoon avocado **or** guacamole

2 cashews

3 olives **or** pistachios

6 peanuts

So a woman may choose to add:

- Olive oil and vinegar dressing (1 teaspoon olive oil plus vinegar to taste) **or**

- 1½ teaspoons almond butter **or**

- 3 macadamia nuts, crushed

A man may want to have:

- Olive oil and vinegar dressing (1⅓ teaspoons olive oil plus vinegar to taste) **or**

- 2 teaspoons almond butter **or**

- 4 macadamia nuts, crushed

Putting It All Together

A woman may choose to eat for lunch:

- 3 ounces of skinless chicken breast, a small side salad topped with ¼ cup chickpeas, 1 apple, and a salad dressing that consists of 1 teaspoon olive oil plus vinegar to taste **or**

- 3 ounces deli meat, 1 piece of string cheese, 1 piece of bread (about 9 grams), 1 cup of blueberries, and 1½ teaspoons of almond butter to spread on the bread **or**

- ¾ cup cottage cheese mixed with 1 cup grapes and ⅓ cup mandarin oranges and 3 macadamia nuts, crushed

A man might choose the following for lunch

- 4 ounces skinless chicken breast, 1 apple, ½ cup chickpeas on top of a side salad, and a dressing that consists of 1⅓ teaspoons olive oil plus vinegar to taste **or**

- 4½ ounces deli meat, 1 piece of string cheese, 1 piece bread, 1 cup blueberries, 1 peach, and 2 teaspoons almond butter to spread on the bread **or**

- 1 cup cottage cheese mixed with 1 cup grapes, ⅔ cup mandarin oranges, and 4 macadamia nuts, crushed

ZONE SALAD BAR SIMPLIFIED

We developed this chart on www.drsears.com, the official Zone Diet website, a couple of years ago. The chart gives a long list of different ingredients that can be used to complete the carbohydrate content of a Zone salad. It tells what to choose at the supermarket or restaurant salad bar to make sure enough carbohydrates are consumed for lunch. Since it takes two heads of iceberg lettuce to equal a block, consider it a free carbohydrate.

For example, a woman, who needs 3 blocks of carbohydrates for lunch, might choose ¼ cup black beans, ¼ cup chickpeas, and ¼ cup hummus to use as a dressing. Add 3 blocks of protein, such as 3 ounces of skinless chicken breast, but don't add any fat blocks, because hummus contains fat. Or perhaps she is in the mood for a salad with lots of vegetables on top. She could top her lettuce with ⅓ cup artichoke hearts, 1 cup broccoli florets, ½ cup sliced celery, and 1 cup chopped mushrooms. That's 1 block. Add a piece of fruit to make it 3. Add 3 blocks of protein and a dressing of 1 teaspoon olive oil plus vinegar, salt, and pepper to taste.

A typical man needs 4 blocks of carbohydrate per meal. For his salad bar carbs, he might choose ⅓ cup water chestnuts and 2 tomatoes and have a fruit salad of ½ apple and ⅓ cup Mandarin oranges for dessert. Add 4 blocks of protein, such as 6 ounces of shrimp and a dressing of 1⅓ teaspoons olive oil plus vinegar, salt and pepper to taste.

Eat 4 of the ingredients below to equal 1 carb block	Eat 1 ingredient below to equal 1 carb block
Artichoke, 1 medium	Black beans, ¼ cup
Artichoke hearts, ⅓ cup	Green beans, 1½ cups
Green beans, ⅓ cup	Chickpeas, ¼ cup
Broccoli florets, 1 cup	Kidney beans, ¼ cup
Cauliflower pieces, 1 cup	Hummus, ¼ cup (also count fat)
Bamboo shoots, 1 cup	Lentils, ¼ cup
Celery, sliced, ½ cup	Tomatoes, 2
Cucumber, sliced, 1 cup	Water chestnuts, 1 cup
Pepper, chopped, ½ cup	Mandarin oranges, ⅓ cup
Mushrooms, chopped, 1 cup	Grapes, ½ cup
Onion, chopped, ⅓ cup	Apple ½
Yellow squash, sliced, ½ cup	
Zucchini, sliced, ½ cup	
Snow peas, ⅓ cup	
Tomato, ½	

Lunch at work will be much more Zoneful if you pack it at home. You can quickly make a lunch using the charts in this chapter. Another good tip is to cook extra protein for dinner the night before or cook a Zone soup or chili, such as the chili on page 120. Pack your lunch in plastic containers so that they can be popped into the microwave at work. The biggest benefit of packing your lunch and following the Zone eating schedule is that you won't be so famished that you chip in for the office pizza run and then wolf down two slices. Remember, one bad carbohydrate leads to another, which means that you may be raiding the vending machine for the rest of the day.

Of course, there will be days when you don't have time to make lunch before you leave for work. There are restaurants everywhere that allow you to stay in the Zone, especially if you know what to look for.

• Stop at a convenience store such as White Hen Pantry for a bowl of beef barley soup and a piece of skinless chicken breast or deli chicken or turkey.

- Get turkey, chicken, and ham at a homestyle chicken restaurant such as Boston Market. Eat two or three Zone sides—creamed spinach, roasted vegetables, and green beans.

- If fast-food restaurants are your only recourse, a chicken Caesar salad and a bowl of chili will keep you in the Zone.

- At Bertucci's or similar Italian restaurants, have the chicken scaloppini and the hummus (without the pita bread).

- At a deli, try a chicken breast sandwich and throw away ½ of the bun.

- Even a pizza with a very thin crust that is loaded with chicken and cheese will do if you eat the crust of the first piece and just the toppings of the other pieces.

- At Dunkin' Donuts choose a ham, egg, and cheese croissant and some vegetable soup.

- Kentucky Fried Chicken offers skinless chicken and green beans. (Bring an apple for dessert.)

- At Taco Bell, have one beef enchilada and a bowl of chili.

Although most frozen dinners aren't totally Zoneful, some can be used in emergencies, such as when the boss buys pork fried rice for everyone. You'll be better able to resist if you have something to fall back on. Here's another "gramming" lesson to help you put a frozen dinner into the Zone.

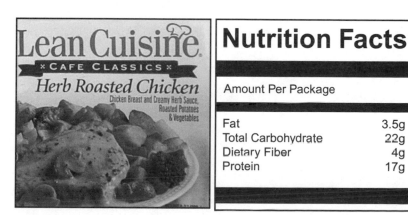

Lean Cuisine's Herb Roasted Chicken, for example, contains 17 grams of protein, 18 grams of carbs, and 3.5 grams of fat. For a woman the protein is close enough. Add a peach and 12 peanuts and you've got a Zone lunch. For men, add a a piece of string cheese, an apple, and 6 cashews.

What do you do when you have to order in for a working meeting? For one thing, don't buy pizza for everyone. You can have a spread with deli meats, vegetables, and a healthful dip. Add some vegetable side dishes from places like Boston Market, including spinach and grilled vegetables. Order a big bowl of hummus with raw veggies and small wedges of pita bread and include a fruit plate for dessert. You'll find your post-lunch work session more productive if everyone eats a Zone lunch.

Lunch at work can be the biggest problem facing Zoners. These simple tips and the following recipes will help solve the problem.

LUNCH RECIPES

Tuna and Spinach Salad with Yogurt-Dill Dressing and Melon-Berry Smoothie

Rachel Albert-Matesz

Prep: 20 minutes   **Yield:**   4 (4-block) meals

For a change of taste, replace the spinach with mesclun, spring greens, endive with escarole, or romaine; replace the tuna with canned salmon, cooked chicken, or turkey breast. For further inspiration, use your favorite herbs instead of dill.

Block Size	Ingredients
Yogurt Dressing	
1 protein, 1 carbohydrate	1 cup organic low-fat yogurt, such as Stonyfield Farms
10 fat	⅓ cup Nayonnaise (soy-based sandwich spread)
2 carbohydrate	4 teaspoons fructose powder
	1 tablespoon Dijon mustard
	¼ cup minced fresh parsley leaves
	1½ teaspoons minced fresh dill weed **or** ⅓ teaspoon dried
	¼ teaspoon finely ground white or black pepper
	Finely ground sea salt (to taste)

Tuna and Spinach Salad

1 carbohydrate	10 cups baby spinach, washed, spun dry
2 carbohydrate	2 medium-size Roma tomatoes, thinly sliced or diced
1 carbohydrate	1 cup bottled artichoke hearts, drained
½ carbohydrate	2 cups English cucumber, peeled, quartered, thinly sliced
¼ carbohydrate	1 cup minced scallions (green onions)
12 protein	12 ounces water packed, no-salt tuna, drained
6 fat	18 lightly toasted walnut halves, coarsely chopped
	¼ cup capers, rinsed and chopped (optional)

Melon Berry Cooler

2 carbohydrate	⅔ cup apple juice
4 carbohydrate	3 cups cubed honeydew or cantaloupe melon
2¼ carbohydrate	1¼ cups fresh, rinsed and drained or thawed frozen blueberries
	1 teaspoon pure vanilla extract
	½ teaspoon ground cinnamon
	6 ice cubes

Instructions

1 Combine the dressing ingredients in a small bowl or wide-mouth 16-ounce jar and whisk or shake well.

2 Layer and divide the salad ingredients among 4 large dinner plates or in 4 (1-quart) bowls with snap-on lids for pack lunches. Toss with the dressing just before serving.

3 Combine the Melon Berry Cooler ingredients in a blender. Cover and process until smooth, then pour into 4 tall glasses or chill in Thermos bottles for meals to go.

Tuna and White Bean Salad

www.drsears.com

Prep: 15 minutes plus 30 minutes to chill   **Yield:** 1 (4-block) meal

Block Size	Ingredients
2 carbohydrate	½ cup canned white beans
4 protein	4 ounces solid white albacore tuna, packed in water
½ carbohydrate	1 large bell pepper, chopped
1 carbohydrate	½ cup minced roasted red pepper
	2 large stalks celery, chopped
½ carbohydrate	¾ cup chopped red onion
4 fat	1⅓ teaspoons olive oil
	3 tablespoons red wine vinegar
	Salt, pepper, and spices (cumin is recommended), to taste

Instructions

Drain and rinse the beans in cold water. In a large bowl, toss all the ingredients together gently so as not to crush the beans. Serve well chilled.

Tuna and White Bean Salad with Arugula, Capers, and Feta and Dill Dressing

Rachel Albert-Matesz

Prep: 15 minutes   **Yield:**   4 (4-block) meals

Look for small bags of prewashed baby arugula leaves (about 3 inches long) in the produce section of natural foods stores and supermarkets. They will be less peppery than long arugula leaves. If you can't find arugula, substitute a spring salad mix or baby greens salad mix.

Block Size	Ingredients
Tuna–White Bean Salad	
½ carbohydrate	5 cups baby arugula, washed, spun dry, and sliced if large
½ carbohydrate	5 cups romaine hearts, washed, dried, and thinly sliced
¼ carbohydrate	⅔ cup scallions (green onions), white part and most of green part, washed, trimmed, and minced
¼ carbohydrate	½ large yellow bell pepper, halved, seeded, and thinly sliced
2 carbohydrate	4 small Roma tomatoes, cut into small wedges
½ carbohydrate	2 cups English cucumber, peeled, quartered, and thinly sliced
8 carbohydrate	2 cups unsalted cooked white beans
12 protein	12 ounces drained, water packed, tuna, preferably unsalted
	¼ cup bottled capers, drained
4 protein	4 ounces feta cheese, crumbled

Dill Dressing

16 fat	1⅔ tablespoons extra-virgin olive oil
1 carbohydrate	⅓ cup orange juice
	2 teaspoons Dijon or roasted garlic mustard
	½ teaspoon red pepper flakes **or** ground black pepper
	2 teaspoon dried dill weed **or** 2 tablespoons fresh, minced
3½ carbohydrate	1¾ cup grapes

Instructions

1 Layer and divide the tuna–white bean salad ingredients among 4 serving plates or containers with lids.

2 Combine the dressing ingredients in a small jar. Cover, shake, and spoon over salads before serving, or divide among 4 small bottles, cover, and refrigerate for pack lunches.

3 Serve the grapes for dessert.

Variation

Replace romaine lettuce with endive and escarole.

Tuna Waldorf Salad with Yogurt, Blue Cheese, and Chive Dressing

Rachel Albert-Matesz

Prep: 20 minutes   **Yield:**   4 (4-block) meals

There are probably as many Waldorf salads as there are people who make them. This one is a complete meal, perfect for a pack lunch or picnic. Mark Bittman, author of *How to Cook Everything,* gets credit for the salad dressing, to which I add chives.

Block Size	Ingredients
Blue Cheese Dressing	
1 protein, 1 carbohydrate	½ cup organic low-fat yogurt; ⅔ cup if yogurt does not contain nonfat dry milk
6 protein	6 ounces crumbled Roquefort or other blue cheese, such as Stilton, Maytag, **or** Gorgonzola
1 carbohydrate	⅓ cup lemon juice
	2 teaspoon freeze-dried chives **or** 2 tablespoons minced fresh
	¼ teaspoon ground black pepper, or to taste
	¼ teaspoon finely ground sea salt (optional)
Tuna Waldorf Salad	
1 carbohydrate	10 cups endive and escarole washed, spun dry, thinly sliced
9 protein	9 ounces drained, water packed, tuna, preferably unsalted
16 fat	48 walnut halves, lightly toasted and crumbled
5 carbohydrate	2½ cups seedless grapes

| 8 carbohydrate | 4 small tart-sweet apples, washed, cored, and diced |
| ½ carbohydrate | Juice of ½ orange |

Instructions

1 To make the dressing, combine the yogurt and blue cheese in a small bowl. Mash with a fork, leaving some lumps in place. Stir in the lemon juice and chives. Add pepper and sea salt if desired.

2 Divide the greens, tuna, walnuts, and grapes among 4 serving plates or containers with snap-on lids. Toss the apple slices with the orange juice and arrange them over the salads.

3 Pour the blue cheese dressing over the salads just before serving or divide it among 4 small bottles, cover, and refrigerate until serving or packing in insulated lunch totes.

Variation

Replace endive and escarole with romaine lettuce.

Chickpea and Tuna Garden Salad with Yogurt-Avocado and Chipotle Dressing

Rachel Albert-Matesz

Prep: 25 minutes   **Yield:**   4 (4-block) meals

The idea for this main-dish salad came from *The Encyclopedia of Foods* and my imagination. For the yogurt avocado dressing, I made minor changes to a recipe from Mark Bittman's culinary bible *How to Cook Everything.*

Block Size	Ingredients
Garden Salad	
¾ carbohydrate	7½ cups romaine hearts, washed, spun dry, and thinly sliced
2 carbohydrate	4 small Roma tomatoes, cut into small wedges
1 carbohydrate	4 cups precut broccoli florets
1 carbohydrate	1 cup shredded carrot
¼ carbohydrate	1 cup thinly sliced fresh or drained, canned mushrooms
8 carbohydrate	2 cups canned, unsalted chickpeas, drained
1 carbohydrate	1½ cups red onion, cut in thin rings or half-moon slices
12 protein	12 ounces drained, water packed tuna, preferably unsalted
3 protein	3 hard-boiled eggs, peeled and quartered or cut into rounds
Yogurt Avocado Dressing	
1 protein, 1 carbohydrate	½ cup organic low-fat yogurt; ⅔ cup if yogurt doesn't contain nonfat milk
16 fat	1 cup cubed avocado

1 carbohydrate	⅓ cup lemon juice
	1 tablespoon minced shallot
	1 garlic clove, chopped
	¼ teaspoon ground chipotle (smoked dried jalapeño), or to taste **or** your favorite hot sauce
	½ teaspoon finely ground sea salt (optional)

Instructions

1 Divide and layer the salad ingredients among 4 large salad plates or in 4 (quart-size) containers with snap-on lids, for packed lunches.

2 Blend the dressing ingredients in a blender or food processor. Taste and adjust the seasonings if needed.

3 Pour the dressing over the salads just before serving or divide it among 4 small bottles, cover, and refrigerate until serving or packing in insulated lunch totes.

Variations

- Replace broccoli with cauliflower.
- Lightly steam or parboil broccoli (or cauliflower) until crisp-tender; plunge into ice water, drain, and add to salad in step 1 above.

French Onion Tuna Salad and Veggie Plate

Rachel Albert-Matesz

Prep: 20 minutes plus 1 hour to chill   **Yield:**   4 (4-block) meals

Look for Fantastic Foods Soup & Dip Recipe Mixes on the health food aisle in your local supermarket.

Block Size	Ingredients
French Onion Dip	
2½ protein, 2½ carbohydrate	1⅔ cups organic low-fat yogurt, such as Stonyfield Farms
16 fat	½ cup low-fat mayonnaise or Nayonnaise (soy-based sandwich spread)
2 carbohydrate	One 1.1-ounce package Fantastic Foods Onion Soup & Dip Recipe Mix
13 protein	13 ounces drained, water-packed, no-salt tuna
Salad	
1 carbohydrate	10 cups baby greens salad mix, washed and spun dry
½ carbohydrate	2 cups peeled, thinly sliced cucumber
½ carbohydrate	1 cup thinly sliced red, yellow, or orange bell pepper
4 carbohydrate	One 16-ounce package baby carrots
6 carbohydrate	3 cups seedless grapes

Instructions

1 Combine the yogurt, mayonnaise, and onion dip mix. Stir well, cover, and refrigerate for at least 1 hour. Mix in the tuna.

2 Divide the salad ingredients among 4 serving plates or containers with snap-on lids. Divide the tuna mixture into 4 portions and spoon over the salad vegetables. Serve immediately or transport in bowls with fitted lids. Serve the grapes for dessert.

Variation

Replace the onion dip mix with garlic herb-flavored dip mix.

Shrimp, Asparagus, and Tomato Salad with White Beans and Goat Cheese

Rachel Albert-Matesz

Prep: 30 minutes   **Yield:**   4 (4-block) meals
Cooking: 15 minutes

I added white beans, artichoke hearts, sun-dried tomatoes, and herbs to Mark Bittman's *Shrimp Salad Mediterranean Style* (from *How to Cook Everything*) to make a complete meal.

Block Size	Ingredients
Shrimp and Vegetables	
	4 cups salt-free chicken stock or broth
12 protein	18 ounces medium-to-large raw shrimp, peeled
	1½ cups filtered water
4 carbohydrate	48 asparagus spears, bottom 1 to 2 inches snapped off and discarded, spears cut into 1-inch pieces
1 carbohydrate	1½ cups red onion, cut into rings
Salad Topping	
1 carbohydrate, 4 fat	8 sun-dried tomato halves packed in olive oil, drained and thinly sliced (Mediterranean Organic brand preferred)
8 carbohydrate	2 cups drained, canned unsalted white beans
6 protein	6 ounces goat cheese, coarsely crumbled
	¼ cup capers, drained

Dressing

1 carbohydrate	Juice of 1 lemon (about ⅓ cup)
12 fat	4 teaspoons extra-virgin olive oil
	2 teaspoons dried, crumbled basil **or**
	2 tablespoons minced fresh basil
	2 garlic cloves, finely minced or pressed
	2 teaspoons dried Italian herb blend,
	crumbled
	Finely ground sea salt and freshly ground
	black pepper

Instructions

1 Bring the stock to boil in large saucepan or deep skillet over medium-high heat. Reduce the heat to medium-low and immediately add the shrimp. Cover and simmer for 2 minutes. Turn off the heat, uncover, cool for 10 minutes, and drain, reserving the stock for another use.

2 Bring the water to boil in a 3-quart saucepan fitted with a collapsible metal steamer or pasta insert. Add the asparagus spears and tips, and onion. Cover and steam until just tender and easily pierced with a fork, 5 to 7 minutes. Plunge the vegetables into a bowl of ice water, drain well, and transfer to a large salad bowl. Add the tomatoes, beans, cheese, and capers. Top with the shrimp.

3 In a medium bowl, whisk together the dressing ingredients. Pour the dressing over the salad and toss to coat. Divide the salad among 4 large serving plates and serve immediately, or cover and chill for 1 to 4 hours.

Variation

Replace the shrimp with 18 ounces of cooked salmon, or 12 ounces of tuna, turkey, or chicken breast.

Spinach Dip with Shrimp and Crudites

Rachel Albert-Matesz

Prep: 20 minutes   **Yield:**   4 (4-block) meals
Cooking: 8 minutes

Fantastic Foods makes the health food equivalent of Lipton Cup-A-Soup and dip mixes that don't contain MSG and other preservatives. They come in four flavors you can use to dress up all sorts of dishes. Keep your freezer stocked with frozen, precooked shrimp for convenience.

Block Size	Ingredients
Spinach Yogurt Dip	
4 protein, 4 carbohydrate	2 cups low-fat organic yogurt; 2⅔ cups if the yogurt does not contain nonfat dry milk
16 fat	½ cup Nayonnaise (soy-based sandwich spread)
2 carbohydrate	One 1.1-ounce package Fantastic Foods Onion **or** Garlic-Herb Soup and Dip Recipe Mix
	10-ounce package frozen cut leaf spinach, thawed and drained
Vegetables and Shrimp	
4 carbohydrate	One 16-ounce package baby carrots
1 carbohydrate	4 cups precut raw cauliflower florets
1 carbohydrate	4 cups precut raw broccoli florets
½ carbohydrate	4 celery stalks, cut into sticks
2 carbohydrate	2 cups cherry tomatoes
12 protein	18 ounces cooked, peeled shrimp
1½ carbohydrate	1½ tangerines

Instructions

1 Combine the dip ingredients in a large bowl. Stir well, cover, and refrigerate for at least 2 hours.

2 Add 1 inch of water to a 3-quart saucepan. Rest a metal folding steamer in the bottom; the water should come to just below the bottom of the steamer. (Alternatively, fill a stockpot with 2 inches of water and add a pasta insert.) Cover and bring to a boil over medium-high heat. Layer the carrots, then the cauliflower, cover, and cook 2 to 3 minutes. Add the broccoli florets, cover, and cook 2 to 6 minutes more, or until the broccoli is bright green and crisp-tender.

3 Plunge the cooked vegetables into a bowl of ice water to stop the cooking and hold the colors. Drain and arrange the vegetables in sections around the outer edges of each of 4 serving plates. Arrange the tomato, celery, and shrimp in a circle inside the vegetables on the plates.

4 Divide the dip among 4 small custard cups. Place 1 custard cup in the center of each serving plate, surrounded by the vegetables and shrimp. Serve the tangerine slices for dessert.

Mediterranean-Style Shrimp and Chickpea Salad

Rachel Albert-Matesz

Prep: 30 minutes   **Yield:**   4 (4-block) meals
Cooking: 3 minutes

Shrimp salad goes from side dish to meal in a bowl in this easy and versatile recipe. If you can't find baby arugula leaves, which are mild in flavor and only a few inches long, use a 50/50 mixture of arugula and romaine, red-leaf, or green-leaf lettuce, or substitute an Italian salad mix (often sold as mesclun, baby, or spring greens).

Block Size	Ingredients
1 carbohydrate	10 cups baby arugula or Italian salad mix, washed, spun dry
	4 cups salt-free chicken stock or broth
16 protein	1½ pounds medium-to-large shrimp, peeled
Salad	
8 carbohydrate	2 cups drained, canned unsalted chickpeas
2 carbohydrate	16 oil-packed sun-dried tomato halves, drained, sliced, oil reserved
2 carbohydrate	1 cup artichoke hearts, bottled or canned, drained
1 carbohydrate	Juice of 1 lemon (about ⅓ cup)
16 fat	5⅓ teaspoons olive oil (from the sun-dried tomatoes)
	½ cup minced fresh parsley
	1 small garlic clove, finely minced
	2 teaspoons dried Italian herb blend, crumbled
	Finely ground sea salt and freshly ground black pepper
2 carbohydrate	1 mini pita pocket, quartered

Instructions

1 Divide the salad greens among 4 large dinner plates or quart-size bowls with snap-on lids.

2 Bring the stock to boil in a large saucepan or deep skillet over medium-high heat. Reduce the heat to medium-low and add the shrimp. Cover and simmer 2 minutes. Turn off the heat, uncover, and cool for 10 minutes.

3 Combine the remaining salad ingredients (except the pita bread) and toss to coat.

4 Drain the shrimp, reserving the stock for another use. Add the shrimp to the bean-vegetable mixture and toss to coat. Taste and add additional sea salt or pepper if desired.

5 Spoon the salad over the 4 greens plates or serving bowls and top with the pita wedges. Serve immediately or cover and refrigerate for later.

Variation

Replace the pita pocket with 2 cups strawberries for dessert.

Chicken and Black Bean Salad with Feta, Artichoke Hearts, and Arugula

Rachel Albert-Matesz

Prep: 20 minutes   **Yield:**   4 (4-block) meals

Arugula adds a slightly spicy kick to green salads. If you can't find it, substitute frisée, escarole, endive, or additional romaine. If you use prewashed salad greens, give them a good rinse, then dry them in a salad spinner.

Block Size	Ingredients
Chicken and Black Bean Salad	
½ carbohydrate	5 cups baby arugula, washed and spun dry, sliced if large
½ carbohydrate	5 cups romaine hearts, washed, dried, and thinly sliced
½ carbohydrate	1 yellow bell pepper, halved,seeded, and diced
2 carbohydrate	4 small Roma tomatoes, cut into small wedges
½ carbohydrate	¾ cup red onion or sweet white onion, cut in thin rings
8 carbohydrate	2 cups no-salt-added, cooked, drained black beans
1 carbohydrate	1 cup bottled artichoke hearts, drained
	¼ cup drained capers
4 protein	4 ounces feta cheese, crumbled
12 protein	12 ounces cooked skinless chicken breast, cut into strips **or** 18 ounces deli-style chicken breast, sliced

Dressing

16 fat	5⅓ teaspoons extra-virgin olive oil
1 carbohydrate	⅓ cup lemon juice
2 carbohydrate	4 teaspoons fructose powder **or**
	1 tablespoon honey
	¼ cup low-sodium chicken stock or broth
	¼ teaspoon guar gum **or** xanthan gum
	2 teaspoons Dijon mustard
	½ teaspoon red pepper flakes **or** ground black pepper
	2 teaspoon dried oregano, crumbled
	2 garlic cloves, minced or pressed
	¼ teaspoon ground black pepper **or** red pepper

Instructions

1 Layer and divide chicken and black bean salad ingredients among 4 serving plates or large bowls with snap-on lids.

2 Combine the dressing ingredients in a small jar. Cover and shake until smooth. Spoon the dressing over the salads just before serving or divide among 4 small bottles, cover, and refrigerate for pack lunches.

Variations

Replace chicken with turkey breast or leftover cooked salmon.

Curried Chicken Waldorf Salad

Rachel Albert-Matesz

Prep: 20 minutes   **Yield:**   4 (4-block) meals

Look for hormone- and antibiotic-free ready-to-eat rotisserie chickens in your local natural foods store or supermarket, or roast a bird on the weekend or cook it overnight on low in a slow cooker.

Block Size	Ingredients
Curried Yogurt Dressing	
2 protein, 2 carbohydrate	1 cup organic low-fat yogurt; 1⅓ cups if yogurt does not contain nonfat dry milk
8 fat	8 teaspoons reduced-fat mayonnaise **or** 4 tablespoons Nayonnaise (soy-based sandwich spread)
2 carbohydrate	4 teaspoons fructose powder
	2 teaspoons curry powder
	2 tablespoons minced fresh parsley or cilantro
Salad	
1 carbohydrate	10 cups romaine hearts, washed, spun dry, and thinly sliced
14 protein	14 ounces cooked chicken breast **or** combination breast and thigh meat, shredded or cut into 1-inch cubes
6 carbohydrate	3 small tart-sweet apples, cored and minced
½ carbohydrate	¾ cup minced Walla Walla Sweet **or** Vidalia onions
½ carbohydrate	2 cups minced celery hearts **or** celery sticks
8 fat	16 cashews, raw **or** lightly toasted, coarsely chopped
4 carbohydrate	4 tablespoons raisins

Instructions

1 In a medium bowl, combine the yogurt, mayonnaise, fructose, curry powder, and parsley or cilantro. Stir and set aside.

2 Divide the salad greens among 4 serving plates or containers with snap-on lids.

3 Combine the remaining ingredients in a medium bowl. Add the yogurt dressing and stir to coat, then spoon over greens and serve.

Variation

Replace romaine lettuce with endive and escarole.

Mex-Chicken Chili

www.drsears.com

Prep: 15 minutes
Cooking: 2 minutes

Yield: 1 (4-block) meal

Block Size	Ingredients
3 protein	3 ounces cooked chicken, cut into 1-inch cubes
1 protein	1 ounce low-fat shredded cheese
2 carbohydrates	½ cup no-salt-added, cooked, drained black beans
1 carbohydrate	½ cup salsa
4 fat	12 black olives, chopped
	Chili powder and/or cayenne pepper to taste
1 carbohydrate	½ orange, sliced

Instructions

Combine all the ingredients except the orange into a microwave-safe bowl and mix. Microwave until hot and serve.

Variation

Add fresh chopped tomatoes, onions, parsley, or cilantro for a bit of added zip.

Turkey, Three Bean, and Artichoke Salad with Ketchup and Basil Dressing

Rachel Albert-Matesz

Prep: 20 minutes   **Yield:**   4 (4-block) servings

The classic three-bean salad goes from side dish to main dish with the addition of diced turkey breast. The idea for the dressing comes from James Peterson's inspiring book, *Simply Salmon,* which I Zoned and jazzed up with herbs and mustard.

Block Size	Ingredients
Salad	
16 protein	16 ounces cooked turkey breast, cut into 1-inch cubes
3 carbohydrate	¾ cup drained, canned unsalted kidney beans
3 carbohydrate	¾ cup drained, canned unsalted chickpeas
2 carbohydrate	½ cup drained, canned unsalted navy beans
1 carbohydrate	2 cups thinly sliced celery (with tops)
½ carbohydrate	¾ cup finely minced red onion
1 carbohydrate	½ cup bottled, roasted sweet peppers, thinly sliced
	½ cup finely minced fresh parsley
1 carbohydrate	1 cup artichoke hearts, bottled or canned, drained, and quartered
Dressing	
3 carbohydrate	6 tablespoons fruit-sweetened ketchup
½ carbohydrate	2 tablespoons balsamic vinegar
16 fat	5⅓ teaspoons olive oil (from the roasted pepper jar)

4 teaspoons dried basil, crumbled, **or**

¼ cup minced fresh basil leaves

2 teaspoons Dijon mustard

1 carbohydrate   10 cups romaine, red leaf, green leaf,

or Italian salad mix, washed and spun dry

Instructions

1 Combine the salad ingredients in a medium bowl.

2 Combine and whisk the dressing ingredients in a small bowl. Pour over the bean mixture and toss to coat. Cover and refrigerate for several hours or overnight, if time permits.

3 Just before serving, divide the salad greens among 4 large dinner plates or quart bowls with snap-on lids. Top with the bean salad and serve.

Variations

Replace turkey with chicken breast, peeled and cooked shrimp, tuna, salmon, or lean pork loin.

Zoned Hummus and Veggie Plate

Rachel Albert-Matesz

Prep: 20 minutes   **Yield:**   4 (4-block) servings

Chickpeas, like other beans, contain far more carbs than protein. Adding tuna creates a better protein-to-carbohydrate ratio. This protein packed dip goes well with vegetables in pack lunches.

Block Size	Ingredients
Hummus	
8 carbohydrate	2 cups drained, canned, cooked chickpeas (save juice)
14 protein	14 ounces drained, canned, no-salt, water-packed tuna
2 protein	2 hard-boiled eggs
16 fat	½ cup raw or toasted, unsalted sesame tahini
1 carbohydrate	⅓ cup fresh lemon juice (1 lemon)
	¼ cup minced fresh parsley
	3 garlic cloves, minced
	1 teaspoon ground cumin
	½ teaspoon ground black pepper
	1 cup chickpea juices or filtered water
	½ teaspoon sea salt (optional)
	Ground paprika, for garnish
Vegetables	
½ carbohydrate	5 cups romaine lettuce **or** baby greens salad mix
½ carbohydrate	2 cups peeled, sliced cucumber
1 carbohydrate	2 tomatoes, sliced

| 1 carbohydrate | 2 cups celery sticks |
| 4 carbohydrate | 2 whole-wheat pita pockets, halved |

Instructions

1 To make the hummus, combine the chickpeas, tuna, eggs, tahini, lemon juice, parsley, garlic, cumin, pepper, and chickpea juices or water in the work bowl of a food processor. Add sea salt if desired. Cover and process until smooth, stopping to scrape down the sides with a spatula. Add additional water as needed to blend. Taste and adjust the seasonings. Divide into 4 containers with lids, garnish with paprika, cover, and refrigerate.

2 Divide the vegetables among 4 containers with lids. Place each pita bread half in a small plastic or wax paper bag. Cover and chill.

3 At lunch, spoon the hummus over the lettuce, tomato, and cucumbers. Stuff a portion of this mixture in a pita half and eat the rest on the side with the celery sticks.

Variation

Replace pita bread with 1 orange and 1 small apple, quartered.

Tropical Delight Fruit Salad with Vanilla Yogurt Sauce

Rachel Albert-Matesz

Prep: 10 minutes   **Yield:**   4 (4-block) meals

Vanilla whey protein powder produces the creamiest texture and taste. If you use unsweetened protein powder or egg white protein, you may need to add additional stevia. Look for
the strawberry, mango, and pineapple fruit blend in your supermarkets' freezer case.

Block Size	Ingredients
Vanilla Yogurt Sauce	
4 protein, 4 carbohydrate	2 cups organic low-fat yogurt; 2⅔ cup if yogurt does not contain nonfat dry milk
16 fat	1 cup low-fat organic sour cream
12 protein	Four 1-ounce scoops vanilla egg white protein **or** whey protein (about 1 cup)
	2 teaspoons pure vanilla extract in a nonalcoholic base **or** 1 teaspoon pure vanilla in alcohol
	2 teaspoons minced bottled ginger root **or** ¼ teaspoon ground ginger, or to taste
	⅛ to ¼ teaspoon stevia extract powder **or** liquid (optional)
Fruit Salad	
4 carbohydrate	4 cups sliced fresh **or** thawed frozen strawberries
4 carbohydrate	1⅓ cups fresh **or** thawed frozen cubed mango
4 carbohydrate	2 cups sliced fresh **or** thawed frozen pineapple
	1 tablespoon finely chopped fresh mint leaves (optional)

Instructions

1 In a small bowl, combine all the yogurt sauce ingredients except the stevia. Stir, taste, and add ⅛ teaspoon stevia if a sweeter taste is desired. Blend, taste, and adjust as needed. Cover and chill for several hours or overnight if time permits.

2 In a large bowl, stir together the fruit and mint. Divide among 4 serving bowls, top with the yogurt mixture, and serve immediately.

Variation

Replace the mango with 1¼ cups drained water-packed Mandarin oranges.

Dinners

One night a couple of years ago, I didn't feel like cooking. I wanted to go out to eat, but Barry wanted to eat at home. Guess who won? My revenge was to plop some soy protein crumbles over a little olive oil in a pan, add a jar of salsa, and stir in a can of black beans. I heated it, sprinkled some grated cheese on top, and called it dinner.

That will show him, I thought.

He thought I had prepared a great-tasting chili, perfectly Zoned. Since that night, we've often eaten the same dish, because it tastes good and makes us feel good, too. Of course, I usually jazz it up with sun-dried tomatoes, onions, green peppers, and spices. You can use all the herbs and spices you want and still stay in the Zone. Or sometimes I return to the original recipe, basically a Zone meal in seconds.

—*Lynn Sears*

In chapter 3, we said that breakfast doesn't necessarily have to feature breakfast foods. The same is true for dinner. A power dinner for me is an egg white omelet and oatmeal. We eat that breakfast for dinner when we have a long night of work ahead of us and need to feel energized.

Put together dinners the same way you put together breakfasts and lunches. Women should choose three protein blocks, three carbohydrate blocks, and three fat blocks. Men should choose four protein blocks, four carbohydrate blocks, and four fat blocks. Again, if you find the idea of blocks confusing, think of selections instead—three protein, carbohydrate, and fat selections for women and four of each for men.

A complete Zone Food Block Guide on page 365 gives countless combinations to use to make Zone meals. Here are a few choices to get you started.

Let's begin with protein.

Women should choose any combination that gives them a total of three blocks of protein.

Men should choose any combination that gives them a total of four.

1 block

1 ounce lean beef (range-fed or game) **or** skinless chicken breast **or** skinless turkey breast **or** freshwater bass **or** sardines **or** tuna canned in water **or** tuna steak **or** low-fat cheese

1½ ounces ground turkey **or** lean ground beef **or** sea bass **or** calamari **or** cod **or** clams **or** crabmeat **or** haddock **or** lobster **or** mackerel **or** salmon **or** shrimp **or** snapper **or** trout

2 ounces firm tofu

7 grams of soy products

That means a woman might choose:

- 3 ounces of skinless chicken breast **or**

- 4½ ounces of scallops **or**

- 4 ounces of tofu (in a stir-fry) with 1 ounce of low-fat grated cheese sprinkled on top right before serving

A man might choose:

- 4 ounces of skinless chicken breast **or**
- 6 ounces of scallops **or**
- 6 ounces of tofu (in a stir-fry) with 1 ounce of grated low-fat cheese sprinkled on top right before serving

Next we add the carbohydrates.

Women should choose any combination that gives a total of three blocks.

Men should choose any combination that gives a total of four.

1 block

⅛ cup dry pearl barley (check label: 1 block is 9 grams)

¼ cup black beans **or** chickpeas **or** kidney beans **or** lentils

⅓ cup water chestnuts **or** unsweetened applesauce **or** Mandarin oranges canned in water or fruit cocktail canned in water

½ cup tomato sauce **or** salsa **or** blueberries **or** boysenberries **or** grapes **or** peaches canned in water **or** cubed pineapple

½ apple **or** grapefruit **or** nectarine **or** orange **or** pear

1 cup artichoke hearts **or** leeks **or** tomato (canned, chopped) **or** raspberries **or** strawberries (chopped fine) **or** spaghetti squash

1 kiwi **or** 1 nectarine **or** 1 peach **or** 1 plum

1½ cups green beans **or** wax beans **or** Brussels sprouts **or** chopped onions **or** snow peas **or** chopped fresh tomatoes

1½ cucumbers

2 cups whole boiled mushrooms **or** diced zucchini **or** chopped bell peppers **or** sliced celery or cherry tomatoes

3 cups cooked broccoli

4 cups cooked cauliflower

That means a women might choose:

- 1 cup spaghetti squash and 1 cup tomato sauce **or**
- 1½ cups cooked green beans and 1 apple **or**
- ¼ cup chickpeas, ⅓ cup water chestnuts, and 1½ cups snow peas

A man might choose:

- 1 cup spaghetti squash, 1 cup tomato sauce, and 1 cup raspberries **or**
- 1½ cups cooked green beans, 1 apple, and 1 breadstick (no more than 9 grams) **or**
- ¼ cup chickpeas, ⅓ cup water chestnuts, 1½ cups snow peas, and 1 peach

The final component is fat.

Women should choose any combination that gives a total of three blocks.

Men should choose any combination that gives a total of four.

1 block
⅓ teaspoon olive oil
½ teaspoon tahini **or** almond butter **or** natural peanut butter
1 teaspoon slivered almonds
1 macadamia nut
1 tablespoon avocado **or** guacamole
2 cashews
3 olives **or** pistachios
6 peanuts

So a woman might choose:

- 9 olives **or**
- 1 tablespoon slivered almonds **or**
- 1 teaspoon olive oil

And a man might choose:

- 9 olives and 6 peanuts **or**
- 4 teaspoons slivered almonds **or**
- 1⅓ teaspoons olive oil

Putting It All Together

So, for dinner, a woman might choose to have:

- 3 ounces of skinless chicken breast, 1 cup spaghetti squash, 1 cup tomato sauce, and 9 chopped olives **or**
- 4½ ounces scallops, 1½ cups cooked green beans topped with 1 tablespoon slivered almonds, and 1 apple **or**
- 4 ounces cubed firm tofu, sautéed in 1 teaspoon of olive oil with ½ cup chickpeas, ⅓ cup water chestnuts, and 1½ cups snow peas, and topped with 1 ounce of low-fat grated cheese.

A man might choose:

- 4 ounces of skinless chicken breast sautéed with 1 cup artichoke hearts, 1 cup tomato sauce, 9 chopped olives, and 6 peanuts, and 1 cup raspberries **or**
- 6 ounces scallops, 1½ cups cooked green beans topped with 4 teaspoons slivered almonds, 1 apple, and 1 breadstick (no more than 9 grams) **or**

- 6 ounces cubed firm tofu, sautéed in 1⅓ teaspoons of olive oil with ¼ cup chickpeas, ⅓ cup water chestnuts, and 1½ cups snow peas, and topped with 1 ounce of low-fat grated cheese, and 1 peach

The recipes in this book cover a lot of different ways to cook dinner in the Zone:

- Making aluminum foil packets for great-tasting meals that are easy to clean up

- Using a slow cooker to make dinner before you leave for work in the morning.

- Cooking soups and stews that taste great for dinner and can be heated up the next day.

- Using barley to offer a counterpoint to vegetables. Think of using barley the way you used to use rice—in stuffed peppers, with beans in a Mexican meal, as a base for "risotto."

- Buying convenience foods to make quick Zone meals.

To create your dinners, use the simple combination charts and recipes in this chapter, the slow-cooking recipes in chapter 9, or the super-fast recipes in chapter 8, "The Can-Do Zone."

DINNER RECIPES

Tuna Burgers with Mango Sauce, Asparagus in Sesame Sauce, and Cherry Cooler

Rachel Albert-Matesz

Prep: 20 minutes   **Yield:**   4 (4-block) servings
Cooking: 10 minutes

For fast healthful food, stock up on frozen tuna and salmon burgers. Read labels; protein and carb blocks vary from one brand to the next. Visit www.beyondfishsticks@aqua-cuisine.com for some very helpful information.

Block Size	Ingredients
Mango Sauce	
1 protein, 1 carbohydrate	½ cup organic, low-fat yogurt, such as Stonyfield Farms
	2 teaspoons peeled, finely minced ginger root **or** 2 teaspoons bottled ginger juice
	⅛ to ¼ teaspoon ground red pepper
3 carbohydrate	1 cup cubed fresh or thawed frozen mango
Asparagus	
4 carbohydrate	48 small to medium asparagus spears, rinsed and drained
1 carbohydrate	1½ cups red onion, cut into thin half-moon slices
Sesame Sauce	
9 fat	1 tablespoon toasted sesame oil
1 carbohydrate	2 teaspoons fructose powder

1 tablespoon tamari soy sauce

3 tablespoons brown rice vinegar

1 to 2 garlic cloves, minced

7 fat   2½ tablespoons toasted sesame seeds

Tuna Burgers

15 protein   6 frozen Aqua Cuisine Tuna Burgers
                  (3.1 ounce each)

Cherry Cooler

⅓ cup sparkling water (plain or flavored)

3 carbohydrate   1½ cups chopped fresh or frozen
                      pineapple

3 carbohydrate   1 cup fresh pitted or frozen unsweetened
                      "sweet" cherries

1 teaspoon peeled minced ginger **or**
    ginger juice, or to taste

4 to 6 ice cubes

Instructions

1 Puree the ingredients for the mango sauce in a blender or food processor. Cover and refrigerate.

2 Bend each asparagus spear 1 to 2 inches from the bottom. It will break off more or less where the tender part ends and the woody part begins. Discard the woody portion. Cut the spears into 1-inch pieces and rest them and the onion on a metal steamer in a 4-quart saucepan over boiling water. Cover and steam for 3 to 5 minutes, or until fork-tender. Drain, rinse with cold water, and drain again. Set aside in a bowl.

3 In a small bowl, mix the sesame sauce and pour over asparagus. Stir and set aside.

4 Preheat the grill or broiler or lightly mist a 12-inch skillet with olive oil spray and warm over medium heat for 3 to 4 minutes. Add the frozen burgers and broil, grill, or sauté for 3 or 4 minutes per side, or until desired doneness.

5 Place the cherry cooler ingredients in a blender. Cover and process until smooth. Pour into 4 tall glasses.

6 Divide the asparagus among 4 large dinner plates. Add 1½ burgers per plate, top with the mango sauce, and serve.

Baked Sea Bass, Squash, and Tomato Bisque, and Arugula, Apple, and Cashew Salad

Rachel Albert-Matesz

Prep: 30 minutes   **Yield:**   4 (4-block) meals
Cooking: 8 to 20 minutes

A well-stocked kitchen will allow you to make this dinner in less than thirty minutes.

Block Size	Ingredients
Squash and Tomato Bisque	
1 carbohydrate	1½ cups minced, thawed frozen onions
	1 tablespoon finely minced fresh **or** bottled ginger root
	1 garlic clove, minced **or** ¼ teaspoon garlic powder
½ carbohydrate	½ cup canned, unsalted tomato puree
	¼ cup unsalted chicken stock, broth, or water
4 carbohydrate	One 10-ounce package Cascadian Farm thawed frozen organic winter squash
1 protein, 1 carbohydrate	¾ cup Edensoy Original Soy Milk, or similar brand
	¼ teaspoon ground black pepper
	2 teaspoons light, white, or sweet miso **or** ¼ teaspoon stevia extract powder **or** sea salt (optional)
Sea Bass	
15 protein	Four 5½-ounce sea bass steaks or fillets
	1 tablespoon Dijon mustard
	2 teaspoons paprika
	½ teaspoon lemon pepper

Arugula, Apple, and Cashew Salad

¼ carbohydrate	4 cups prewashed arugula, washed and spun dry
½ carbohydrate	5 cups romaine hearts, washed, spun dry, and finely sliced
¾ carbohydrate	1¼ cups minced celery or celery hearts
4 carbohydrate	¼ cup raisins
7 fat	14 cashews, broken in half
4 carbohydrate	2 small tart-sweet apples, cored, peeled, and thinly sliced

Dressing

9 fat	1 tablespoon extra-virgin olive oil
	2 tablespoons low-sodium chicken broth **or** filtered water
	3 tablespoons organic red wine vinegar **or** brown rice vinegar
	2 teaspoons umeboshi vinegar **or** tamari soy sauce (optional)

Instructions

1 To make the bisque, place the onions, ginger, garlic, tomato, stock, and squash in a medium saucepan. Cover and bring to a low boil over medium heat. Reduce the heat and simmer 20 minutes, or until the squash is tender and the soup has thickened.

2 Preheat the oven to 350° F for ½-inch-thick fillets and 375° F for thicker fillets. Arrange the fish on a 10-inch cake pan or oblong pan lined with parchment paper. In a small bowl, mix the mustard, paprika, and lemon pepper. Spread the mixture over the fish and bake the fish 8 to 10 minutes for ½-inch fillets or 15 to 20 minutes for fillets up to 1 inch thick, or until a knife penetrates with little or no resistance and the flesh is nearly opaque throughout.

3 Layer the salad ingredients in a large bowl. Mix the dressing ingredients in a small jar and toss with salad.

4 Stir the soy milk into the bisque. Puree the bisque in a blender or food processor if desired, then season with pepper, and miso if desired. Pour into 4 soup bowls and serve with fish and salad.

Cider-simmered Salmon with Onion Relish and Broccoli with Sun-Dried Tomatoes

Rachel Albert-Matesz

Prep: 20 minutes   **Yield:**   4 (4-block) meals
Cooking: 20 minutes

Start with precut broccoli and mushrooms, frozen minced onions, and oil-packed sun-dried tomatoes and you can assemble this balanced meal in even less time.

Block Size	Ingredients
Onion Relish	
3 carbohydrate	1 cup apple cider or apple juice
1 carbohydrate	2 teaspoons fructose powder
2 carbohydrate	3 cups finely minced fresh or thawed frozen onions
	3 tablespoons apple cider vinegar
	½ teaspoon sea salt
	2 teaspoons Dijon **or** yellow mustard
16 protein	1½ pounds center-cut salmon fillets, cut into 4 pieces
Vegetables	
2 carbohydrate	8 cups broccoli, cut into bite-size florets
½ carbohydrate	1 yellow bell pepper, halved, seeded, and thinly sliced
½ carbohydrate	2 cups thinly sliced mushrooms

Sun-Dried Tomato Dressing

1⅓ carbohydrate, 6 fat	12 oil-packed sun-dried tomatoes, drained and thinly sliced (Mediterranean Organic brand preferred)
10 fat	1 tablespoon plus ⅛ teaspoon extra-virgin olive oil
	1 tablespoon tamari soy sauce
	2 tablespoons organic red wine vinegar
	1 to 2 garlic cloves, finely minced or pressed
	1 teaspoon dried ground rosemary
	¼ teaspoon ground black pepper, or to taste

Cantaloupe with Berries

2 carbohydrate	½ cantaloupe (5-inch diameter), seeded
3⅓ carbohydrate	1¾ cup blueberries, rinsed and drained

Instructions

1 Combine the onion relish ingredients in a 10- to 12-inch skillet. Rinse the salmon and add it to skillet. Cover and bring to a boil over medium-high heat. Reduce the heat to medium and simmer for 8 to 11 minutes, or until a thin-bladed knife inserts easily into the fish and the flesh is a uniform color throughout. Transfer the fish to serving plates, cover the skillet, and simmer 10 to 12 minutes.

2 Meanwhile, layer the vegetables on a rack in a pot over 2 inches of boiling filtered water. Cover and cook until crisp-tender, 6 to 8 minutes. Mix the sun-dried tomato dressing ingredients in a medium nonmetallic bowl. Drain the vegetables and toss with the dressing.

3 Uncover the onion relish and simmer until it is reduced to a thick sauce. Spoon the sauce over the salmon and serve with the vegetables.

4 Fill the melon half with fruit; cut into quarters at the table, and serve it for dessert.

Salmon with Mustard and Tarragon and White Beans with Capers and Greens

Rachel Albert-Matesz

Prep: 20 minutes plus several hours to chill   **Yield:**   4 (4-block) meals
Cooking: 8 to 20 minutes

Assemble the white bean salad the day or night before serving to allow the flavors to mingle. Cook the salmon just before serving or make it the night before, so it's ready for pack lunches or dinner in a dash. In a pinch, replace the fresh salmon with drained water-packed salmon.

Block Size	Ingredients
White Bean Salad	
8 carbohydrate	2 cups unsalted cooked, drained white beans
1 carbohydrate	2 cups red cherry tomatoes, halved
½ carbohydrate	1 yellow bell pepper, halved, seeded, and finely chopped
½ carbohydrate	¾ cup minced red **or** Walla Walla sweet **or** Vidalia onion
	¼ cup minced fresh parsley leaves
	¼ cup minced fresh basil leaves
	¼ cup bottled capers, drained
1 carbohydrate	⅓ cup lemon juice
16 fat	5⅓ teaspoons extra-virgin olive oil
	Freshly ground black pepper and sea salt, to taste
Salmon	
16 protein	1½ pounds center-cut salmon fillets, cut into 4 pieces
½ carbohydrate	2½ tablespoons lemon juice

2 teaspoons Dijon mustard

2 teaspoons dried tarragon

Sparkling Grape Juice

4 carbohydrate

1⅓ cups red grape juice, chilled

⅔ cup sparkling mineral water, chilled

½ carbohydrate

5 cups baby arugula or assorted salad greens, washed and spun dry, thinly sliced if large

Instructions

1 In a medium bowl, combine the white bean salad ingredients and toss to coat. Taste and adjust the seasonings as desired. Cover and refrigerate for several hours or overnight.

2 Preheat the oven or toaster oven to 350°F for ½-inch thick salmon fillets, 375°F for thicker fillets. Line a 13 x 9 x 2-inch or 11 x 9-inch shallow baking pan with unbleached parchment paper. Rinse the salmon, pat it dry, and place it in the prepared baking pan. In a small bowl, whisk together the lemon juice, mustard, and tarragon and spread it over the salmon. Bake 8 to 10 minutes for ½-inch-thick fillets or 15 to 20 minutes for ½- to 1-inch thick pieces, or until firm to the touch, a knife penetrates with little resistance, or the flesh is a uniform color throughout.

3 In a pitcher, mix the grape juice and mineral water and divide among 4 wine goblets. Divide the greens among 4 large salad plates and top with the white bean salad. Arrange the salmon next to salad and serve.

Variation

If using canned salmon, toss it with the white bean salad before serving.

Salmon Burgers and Asparagus-Chive Relish with Curried Squash Bisque

Rachel Albert-Matesz

Prep: 30 minutes or less   **Yield:** 4 (4-block) meals
Cooking: 20 minutes

Frozen salmon burgers are a great convenience food to have on hand. Look for them in natural foods markets or the health food freezer section of your local supermarket.

Block Size	Ingredients
Squash Bisque	
½ carbohydrate	¾ cup minced thawed frozen onions
	2 teaspoons finely minced fresh or bottled ginger root
	1¼ teaspoons curry powder
	½ cup low-sodium chicken stock
4 carbohydrate	One 10-ounce package Cascadian Farm thawed frozen organic winter squash
1 protein, 1 carbohydrate	¾ cup Edensoy Original Soy Milk or similar brand
	¼ teaspoon ground black pepper
	¼ teaspoon stevia extract powder **or** sea salt
Chive Relish	
12 fat	½ cup Nayonnaise (soy-based sandwich spread)
	3 tablespoons minced, fresh **or** 1 teaspoon dried chives
	½ teaspoon lemon pepper **or** ¼ teaspoon black pepper

2 tablespoons Cascadian Farms Dill Relish
or capers

Asparagus and Salmon

4 carbohydrate	48 asparagus spears, bottom 1 or 2 inches snapped off and discarded, spears cut into 1-inch pieces
15 protein	Six 3.2-ounce Omega Foods Salmon Burgers, frozen
	2 cups filtered water

Fruit Salad

2 carbohydrate	2 tangerines or clementines, peeled and sectioned
2 carbohydrate	1 cup seedless red grapes
2 carbohydrate	1½ cups honeydew melon balls or cubes
½ carbohydrate	2½ tablespoons balsamic vinegar
4 fat	12 pecans or walnuts, lightly toasted and coarsely chopped

Instructions

1 To make the bisque, place the onions, ginger, curry, chicken stock, and squash in a medium saucepan. Cover, bring to a low boil over medium heat, reduce the heat, and simmer for 20 minutes, or until the squash is tender and the soup has thickened.

2 In a small bowl, mix the Nayonnaise, chives, pepper, and dill relish or capers. Cover and chill.

3 Add water and a collapsible metal steamer or pasta insert to a 2- to 3-quart saucepan. Cover, bring to a boil over medium heat, and add cut asparagus spears, then tips. Cover and steam until the asparagus is tender and easily pierced with a fork, 5 to 7 minutes.

4 Lightly mist a 12-inch nonstick skillet or griddle with olive oil. Cook the burgers over medium heat for 2 to 3 minutes per side. Do not overcook. Arrange the burgers and vegetables on 4 serving plates.

5 Stir the soy milk into the bisque. Season with pepper and stevia or salt. Pour into 4 bowls.

6 Combine the fruit and vinegar in a medium bowl. Toss, divide among 4 serving plates, and garnish with the nuts. Top the burgers and/or vegetables with the chive relish and serve with the bisque. Serve the fruit salad for dessert.

Salmon and Apricot Tagine with Spinach in a Spicy Walnut Sauce

Rachel Albert-Matesz

Prep: 40 minutes   **Yield:**   4 (4-block) meals
Cooking: 20 to 25 minutes

This four-star recipe requires more prep time than most of the others in this book, but it's worth the effort. The contrasting flavors, textures, and aromas make this a perfect meal for company or a special evening at home.

Block Size	Ingredients
Spicy Walnut Sauce	
10 fat	30 walnut halves, lightly toasted and coarsely chopped
	½ teaspoon finely ground sea salt
	¼ cup brown rice vinegar **or** apple cider vinegar
	2 teaspoons dried dill weed
	2 cloves garlic, minced or pressed
	½ to 1 teaspoon hot sauce **or** harissa (Moroccan hot sauce) to taste
Apricot Tagine	
6 fat	2 teaspoons extra-virgin olive oil
1 carbohydrate	1½ cups minced onion
	⅔ cup filtered water or chicken stock **or** broth
4 carbohydrate	¼ cup raisins
4 carbohydrate	12 whole, sulfite-free dried Turkish apricots, quartered
	½ teaspoon finely ground sea salt

1 garlic clove, minced

½ teaspoon ground cumin

¼ teaspoon ground white pepper

1 cinnamon stick

1 teaspoon peeled, minced fresh ginger root

   or 1 teaspoon bottled ginger juice

16 protein   1½ pounds center-cut salmon fillets, cut
               into 4 pieces

Spinach

2 carbohydrate   Two 1-pound bags washed, stemmed,
                   trimmed spinach leaves

1 carbohydrate   4 cups thinly sliced mushrooms

4 carbohydrate   4 kiwi fruit, peeled and halved

Instructions

1 Process the walnut sauce ingredients in a food processor or an oversize mortar and pestle.

2 For the apricot tagine, in a 10- to 12-inch skillet over medium heat, heat the oil. Add the onion and sauté until tender, 5 to 7 minutes. Add the remaining apricot tagine ingredients, then the salmon. Cover, bring to a low boil, reduce the heat, and simmer until the salmon is easily pierced with a thin-bladed knife and is a uniform color throughout, 8 to 11 minutes. Transfer the fish to 4 serving plates. Cover the skillet; simmer for 10 to 12 minutes, uncover, and cook away the liquid until the sauce is the desired consistency. Spoon the sauce over the fish.

3 Meanwhile, add the spinach, mushrooms, and ½ cup water to a 3- to 4-quart saucepan. Cover, bring to a boil over medium-low heat, and steam until tender, about 5 minutes. Drain well and toss with the spicy walnut sauce. Divide among the dinner plates. Serve the kiwi for dessert.

Shrimp and Vegetables with Garlic-Herb Dip

Rachel Albert-Matesz

Prep: 20 minutes
Cooking: 8 minutes

Yield: 4 (4-block) meals

Fantastic Foods makes soup and dip mixes without MSG and other preservatives. They come in four flavors you can use to dress up all sorts of dishes. Keep your freezer stocked with frozen, precooked shrimp for convenience.

Block Size	Ingredients
Garlic-Herb Dip	
2½ protein, 2½ carbohydrate	1¼ cups organic low-fat yogurt, such as Stonyfield Farms
16 fat	½ cup low-fat mayonnaise **or** Nayonnaise (soy-based sandwich spread)
2 carbohydrate	One 1.1-ounce package Fantastic Foods Garlic-Herb Soup & Dip Recipe Mix
Shrimp and Vegetables	
	1 to 2 cups filtered water
4 carbohydrate	1⅓ cups water chestnuts
1 carbohydrate	4 cups precut raw cauliflower florets
1 carbohydrate	4 cups precut raw broccoli florets
2 carbohydrate	2 cups cherry tomatoes
14 protein	21 ounces cooked, peeled shrimp
4 carbohydrate	4 tangerines, peeled and sectioned

Instructions

1 In a medium bowl, combine the ingredients for the Garlic-Herb dip. Stir well, cover, and refrigerate at least 1 hour.

2 Add 1 inch of water to a 3-quart saucepan. Rest a metal accordion steamer in the bottom; the water should come to just below the bottom of the steamer. Or, fill a stock pot with 2 inches of water and add a pasta insert. Bring to a boil over medium-high heat. Layer in the water chestnuts, then the cauliflower. Cover and cook 2 to 3 minutes. Add the broccoli florets, cover, and cook 2 to 6 minutes, or until the broccoli is bright green and crisp-tender.

3 Plunge the vegetables into a large bowl of ice water to stop the cooking and hold the color. Drain and arrange the vegetables in sections around the outer edges of each of 4 serving plates. Arrange the tomatoes and cooked shrimp in a circle inside the vegetables on the plates.

4 Divide the garlic-herb dip among 4 small custard cups. Place 1 custard cup in the center of each serving plate, surrounded by the vegetables. Serve with the tangerine slices for dessert.

Variation

Replace garlic-herb dip mix with onion-flavored dip mix.

Ostrich Burgers with Oven Fries and Mixed Vegetables

Rachel Albert-Matesz

Prep: 20 minutes or less   **Yield:**   4 (4-block) meals
Cooking: 15 to 20 minutes

Look for ostrich burgers in the frozen foods section of your local natural foods store and supermarket. Be careful not to cook them too long—they're lean and easily overcooked.

Block Size	Ingredients
Oven Fries	
4 carbohydrate, 8 fat	A little more than half of a 16-ounce package Cascadian Farms Organic French Fries
Salad	
1 carbohydrate	10 cups baby greens or mesclun
1 carbohydrate	2 cups celery hearts or sticks, finely sliced
2 carbohydrate	2 tangerines or clementines, peeled and sectioned
4 fat	8 lightly toasted pecan or walnut halves, coarsely chopped
Burgers	
16 protein	Four 4-ounce thawed frozen ostrich burgers
4 fat	4 tablespoons Nayonnaise (soy-based sandwich spread) **or** low-fat mayonnaise
2 carbohydrate	¾ cup Annie's Naturals No-Fat Yogurt Dressing
4 carbohydrate	2 cups salsa

Instructions

1 Preheat the oven to 425°F. Scatter the fries one layer deep on a baking sheet. Bake 15 to 18 minutes, turning the fries after 10 minutes, to desired color and crispness.

2 Divide the greens, celery, tangerines or clementines, and pecans or walnuts among 4 large salad plates.

3 Lightly mist a large nonstick skillet with cooking spray and warm over medium-high heat. Add the burgers and cook for 2 to 3 minutes per side, until warm and cooked through but slightly pink inside.

4 Divide the burgers and fries among 4 large dinner plates. Top each burger with a tablespoon of Nayonnaise (soy-based sandwich spread) or low-fat mayonnaise. Add the yogurt dressing to the salads. Spoon the salsa over the burgers or fries and serve.

Broiled Chicken Salad with Blue Cheese, Cherries, Pears, and Pecans

Rachel Albert-Matesz

Prep: 40 minutes   **Yield:**   4 (4-block) servings
Cooking: 3 to 5 minutes

Don't let the prep time put you off; the sensuous flavors and textures will more than make up for your investment! If you're pressed for time, start with chicken you've baked, broiled, or grilled in advance. The meat will taste just as good served cold as warm.

Block Size	Ingredients
Salad	
1 carbohydrate	10 cups mixed salad greens, baby greens, or spring mix
1 carbohydrate	2 cups thinly sliced celery, including any green tops
4 protein	4 ounces blue cheese, crumbled
4 carbohydrate	¼ cup dried cherries
4 fat	8 pecan halves, lightly toasted and coarsely chopped
Chicken and Pears	
4 carbohydrate	2 ripe but firm pears or Asian pear-apples, washed, halved, cored, and thinly sliced
½ carbohydrate	Juice of ½ lemon
12 protein	Two 6-ounce skinless chicken breast fillets
	¼ teaspoon ground black pepper
	Sea salt (optional)

Dressing

12 fat	1 tablespoon plus 1 teaspoon unrefined walnut oil
1 carbohydrate	⅓ cup fresh orange juice (from about 1 medium orange)
	2 tablespoons red wine vinegar
	1 tablespoon Dijon mustard

Dessert

2 carbohydrate	2 tangerines, peeled and sectioned
2 carbohydrate	1 cup blueberries, washed and drained
½ carbohydrate	1 teaspoon fructose powder
	½ teaspoon finely grated ginger **or** bottled ginger juice

Instructions

1 On 4 dinner plates, layer the salad ingredients in the order listed. In a medium bowl, toss the pears with the lemon juice and arrange over the salads.

2 Preheat the broiler. Season the chicken breasts with pepper and sea salt, if desired, and lightly mist them with olive oil. Place the chicken on the broiler rack and broil about 6 inches from the heat source, turning once, until cooked through, 3 to 4 minutes per side.

3 Meanwhile, put the dressing ingredients in a small jar, cover, and shake.

4 In a medium bowl, combine the dessert ingredients, tossing to coat. Divide among 4 serving cups.

5 Transfer the cooked chicken to a cutting board. Slice thin, arrange over the salads, and top with the dressing. Serve with the fruit salad.

Slow-Cooked Chicken in Tangerine-Tomato Sauce with Spinach, Pine Nuts, and Currants

Rachel Albert-Matesz

Prep: 25 minutes   **Yield:**   4 (4-block) meals
Cooking: 6 to 7 hours

I made a few modifications to Zone a chicken recipe from *The Best Slow Cooker Cookbook Ever* by Natalie Haughton. To get zest from a tangerine, wash it, then grate only the bright orange part, not the bitter white part. Divide the zest into two portions, one to cook in the stew, the other to add before serving.

Block Size	Ingredients
Chicken	
16 protein	16 ounces skinless boneless chicken thighs, cut into 1½-inch pieces
1 carbohydrate	7 ounces canned diced, peeled, unsalted tomatoes
	Grated zest of 1 large tangerine, divided
1 carbohydrate	Juice of 1 tangerine **or** ½ large orange
1 carbohydrate	4 tablespoons unsalted tomato paste
½ carbohydrate	¾ cup diced red or white onion
2 carbohydrate	½ pound baby carrots, halved or cut in thirds
	1½ teaspoons crumbled dried basil
	1½ teaspoons crumbled dried thyme
	1½ teaspoons crumbled dried oregano
	2 garlic cloves, minced or pressed
1 carbohydrate	2 teaspoons fructose powder
½ carbohydrate	Juice of ½ lemon
	½ teaspoon ground black pepper
3 carbohydrate	3 tangerines, peeled, seeded, and sectioned

Spinach

2 carbohydrate	Two 1-pound bags washed, stemmed, and trimmed spinach leaves
	½ teaspoon finely ground sea salt
7 fat	2⅓ teaspoons extra-virgin olive oil
9 fat	¼ cup (about 1 ounce) pine nuts
	2 garlic cloves, finely minced
3 carbohydrate	3 tablespoons currants
	½ teaspoon finely ground black pepper or lemon pepper

Instructions

1 Combine the chicken, tomatoes, half the tangerine zest, tangerine or orange juice, tomato paste, onion, carrots, basil, thyme, oregano, and garlic in a 3½-quart slow cooker. Cover and cook on LOW for 6 to 7 hours, until the chicken is tender and done.

2 About 15 minutes before serving, wash the spinach in a bowl and drain but do not dry. Coarsely chop the spinach and add it to a large skillet or 4-quart saucepan. Sprinkle with the salt. Cover and cook over medium heat until wilted, about 5 minutes, then drain well.

3 Heat the oil in a dry 12- to 14-inch skillet or 4-quart saucepan. Add the pine nuts, stir, and cook for 2 minutes. Add the garlic, stir for ½ to 1 minute, then add the spinach, currants, and pepper. Cook, stirring frequently, for about 5 minutes. Divide the spinach among 4 salad plates.

4 Stir the fructose, lemon juice, pepper, and remaining half of the tangerine zest into the chicken. Ladle the chicken mixture into 4 shallow soup bowls. Arrange the tangerine sections around each bowl. Serve with the spinach.

Chicken Kali

www.drsears.com

Prep: 15 minutes   **Yield:** 1 (3-block) meals
Cooking: 7 to 8 minutes

Block Size	Ingredients
1 block fat	⅓ teaspoon olive oil
3 blocks protein	3 ounces boneless, skinless chicken breast, cut into strips
½ block carbohydrate	¾ cup chopped Vidalia onion
	1 teaspoon minced garlic, or to taste
	1 teaspoon ground ginger, or to taste
	1 teaspoon mild curry powder, or to taste
	1 teaspoon dried mint, or to taste
½ block carbohydrate	1 red bell pepper, chopped
2 blocks carbohydrate	1 cup pineapple chunks packed in juice, drained
2 blocks fat	2 teaspoons slivered almonds

Instructions

In a wok or sauté pan over high heat, heat the olive oil. Stir-fry the chicken and onion until the chicken is cooked through, about 5 minutes. Sprinkle the chicken mixture with spices to taste. Add the pepper and pineapple and stir-fry just until heated through. Add the almond slivers just before serving.

Chicken and Chickpea Loaf with Brussels Sprouts and Cheese

Rachel Albert-Matesz

Prep: 20 minutes **Yield:** 4 (4-block) servings
Cooking: 60 to 75 minutes

Chicken and chickpeas pair up to make this produce and protein-rich loaf.

Block Size	Ingredients
Chicken and Chickpea Loaf	
2 protein	2 whole eggs **or** 4 egg whites
3 carbohydrate	¾ cup cooked chickpeas
	2½ teaspoons poultry seasoning
	¼ teaspoon ground black pepper
	½ teaspoon sea salt (optional)
10 protein	15 ounces lean ground chicken
2 carbohydrate	⅓ cup non-instant rolled oats, uncooked
1 carbohydrate	2 cups minced celery
½ carbohydrate	1 cup minced yellow or red bell pepper
2 carbohydrate	2 tablespoons dried onion flakes
2 carbohydrate	1 cup no-salt tomato sauce, divided
	1 tablespoon prepared mustard
Brussels Sprouts	
	½ cup filtered water
2½ carbohydrate	One 16-ounce bag frozen Brussels sprouts
10 fat	30 pitted black olives, chopped
4 protein	4 ounces shredded, low-fat Muenster, Jack, or Swiss cheese (1 cup)
	Black pepper, to taste

Fruit Salad

1 carbohydrate	1 tangerine, peeled and sectioned
1 carbohydrate	1 plum, halved, pitted, and cut into wedges
1 carbohydrate	½ cup seedless green grapes
6 fat	18 pecan halves, lightly toasted

Instructions

1 Preheat the oven to 350°F. Mist a 9 x 5-inch loaf pan with olive oil spray.

2 Combine the eggs, chickpeas, and spices in a food processor or blender. Cover, blend until smooth, and pour into a 2-quart mixing bowl. Add the chicken, oats, celery, bell pepper, onion, and ½ cup of the tomato sauce. Mix with clean bare hands and press into the loaf pan. In a small bowl, mix remaining ½ cup tomato sauce and mustard and spread it over the loaf.

3 Bake uncovered for 1 to 1¼ hours, or until the loaf is firm to the touch, pulls away from the sides of the pan, and an instant-read thermometer registers 180°F.

4 Bring the water to boil over medium-low heat in a 1½-quart saucepan. Add the Brussels sprouts, cover, return to a boil, reduce the heat, and simmer 8 to 10 minutes or until tender, stirring occasionally. Drain and sprinkle with the olives and cheese and season with pepper. Cover for 2 to 3 minutes and transfer to 4 serving plates.

5 Cut the loaf into 8 slices. Divide among the 4 plates and serve immediately.

6 Toss the fruit with the nuts and serve for dessert.

Turkey and Blue Cheese Burgers with Spinach and Sun-Dried Tomato Dressing

Rachel Albert-Matesz

Prep: 30 minutes
Cooking: 7 to 9 minutes

Yield: 4 (4-block) servings

The idea for the burgers came from *Meat on the Grill* by David Barich and Thomas Ingalls. The inspiration for the sun-dried tomato dressing came from *George Foreman's Big Book of Grilling, Barbecue and Rotisserie.*

Block Size	Ingredients
Dressing	
1 carbohydrate, 4 fat	8 sun-dried tomato halves packed in olive oil and drained (Mediterranean Organic brand preferred)
	1 garlic clove
1 carbohydrate, 1 protein	½ cup organic low-fat yogurt; ⅔ cups if yogurt does not contain nonfat dry milk
12 fat	⅓ cup plus 1 tablespoon Nayonnaise (soy-based sandwich spread)
	1 tablespoon fresh lemon juice
	¼ teaspoon ground black pepper, or to taste
	½ teaspoon ground rosemary
	Sea salt to taste (optional)
Salad	
½ carbohydrate	5 cups baby spinach, rinsed and spun dry
2 carbohydrate	2 sweet yellow bell pepper, halved, seeded, and diced
½ carbohydrate	¾ cup minced red onion
	¼ cup drained capers

Burgers

11 protein	1 pound plus ½ ounce ground turkey
4 protein	4 ounces blue cheese, crumbled
	4 green onions (scallions), minced
	¼ teaspoon ground black pepper

Dessert

8 carbohydrate	6 cups cubed, seedless watermelon **or**
	2 large slices watermelon (each 10 inches in diameter by 1-inch thick), halved

Instructions

1 Preheat the broiler or grill.

2 Mince the sun-dried tomatoes and garlic in a food processor. Add the remaining dressing ingredients and pulse to combine. Taste and add salt if desired. Scrape into a bowl, cover, and refrigerate.

3 Layer the spinach, pepper, onion, and capers on 4 large dinner plates.

4 Break the turkey into pieces and spread it on a meat-designated cutting board or platter. Sprinkle with the blue cheese, green onions, and pepper. Gently work the seasonings into the meat with your fingers. Form into 4 patties, being careful not to pack the meat too tightly or the burgers will be tough.

5 Broil or grill the burgers 3½ to 4½ minutes per side, or until the juices run clear when pricked with a fork and meat is a uniform color throughout. Be careful not to overcook the meat or it will be dry. Serve the burgers with the salad and sun-dried tomato dressing, with watermelon for dessert.

Turkey Burgers with Chili Powder, Spicy Slaw, and Fruit Salad

Rachel Albert-Matesz

Prep: 20 to 30 minutes plus   **Cooking:** 10 minutes
                1 hour to stand   **Yield:**   4 (4-block) servings

Presliced cabbage saves time; just be sure to wash it. Salting and crushing the cabbage breaks down the fibers and release extra water to yield more tender, flavorful, and digestible coleslaw.

Block Size	Ingredients
Spicy Slaw	
2 carbohydrate	6 cups shredded cabbage, rinsed and drained
½ carbohydrate	½ cup shredded carrot
½ carbohydrate	¾ cup finely minced purple onion
½ carbohydrate	1 cup finely minced celery
	1 rounded teaspoon sea salt
Smoky-Yogurt Dressing	
1 protein,1 carbohydrate	½ cup organic low-fat yogurt, such as Stonyfield Farms
9 fat	1 tablespoon unrefined peanut oil
	1 teaspoon dry mustard
	¼ teaspoon ground chipotle (smoked dried jalapeño pepper)
	1 garlic clove, finely minced or pressed
7 fat	42 lightly roasted peanuts, coarsely chopped
Turkey Burgers	
14 protein	1½ pounds lean ground turkey
1 protein	1 whole egg **or** 2 egg whites

2 carbohydrate

2 tablespoons dried onion flakes

1 tablespoons chili powder

½ teaspoon ground cumin

1 garlic clove, minced or pressed (optional)

½ teaspoon finely ground sea salt **or**

  1 tablespoon tamari

Fruit Salad

4 carbohydrate   3 cups cantaloupe cubes or balls

2 carbohydrate   2 kiwi fruit, peeled, quartered, and thinly
                                          sliced

3½ carbohydrate   1¾ cups seedless red grapes

Instructions

1 Combine the slaw vegetables in a large mixing bowl. Rub and knead the salt into the vegetables with your hands until the cabbage starts to shrink, turns translucent around the edges, and releases water, about 5 minutes. Leave the slaw vegetables at room temperature for 1 hour or chill for several hours.

2 Squeeze the slaw vegetables to release moisture and drain well in a fine mesh strainer. Place the vegetables in a medium bowl. In a small bowl, mix the yogurt, oil, mustard, chipotle, and garlic. Toss the dressing with the slaw vegetables and peanuts. Chill.

3 Break the meat apart in a bowl and add the remaining burger ingredients. Toss with clean bare hands to mix evenly. Divide the mixture into 4 equal portions, then pat into ¾- to 1-inch-thick patties.

4 Mist a 10- to 12-inch heavy-bottomed stainless steel or cast-iron skillet or grill pan with oil. Warm over medium-high heat for 3 to 4 minutes. Add the patties and cook 4 to 5 minutes per side, turning once, until the meat is a uniform color throughout.

5 Mix the fruit salad ingredients together. Serve with the spicy slaw and fruit.

Zoned Bean and Meat Loaf with Cheesy Vegetables and Grape-Nut Mix

Rachel Albert-Matesz

Prep: 20 minutes
Cooking: 60 to 75 minutes

Yield: 4 (4-block) servings

A well-stocked kitchen will make it easy to assemble this hearty dinner. Rolled oats stand in for bread crumbs and the beans make a fiber-rich filler in this remake of the classic meat loaf.

Block Size	Ingredients
Bean and Meat Loaf	
2 protein	2 whole eggs **or** 4 egg whites
3 carbohydrate	¾ cup cooked kidney beans **or** other beans, drained
	1 tablespoon dried, crumbled Italian herb blend
	½ teaspoon ground black **or** red pepper
	1 tablespoon tamari soy sauce (optional)
10 protein	15 ounces lean ground beef
2 carbohydrate	⅓ cups non-instant rolled oats, uncooked
2 carbohydrate	2 tablespoons dried onion flakes
¼ carbohydrate	½ cup minced yellow or red bell pepper
¼ carbohydrate	½ cup minced celery
	¾ teaspoon garlic powder
2 carbohydrate	1 cup low-salt **or** no-salt tomato sauce, divided
Cheesy Vegetables	
	½ cup filtered water
1½ carbohydrate	One 16-ounce bag Bird's Eye frozen broccoli and cauliflower with carrots

	1 tablespoon freeze dried chives **or**
	3 tablespoons minced fresh chives
4 protein	4 ounces grated low-fat Muenster, Jack, **or**
	cheddar cheese

Dessert

5 carbohydrate	2½ cups seedless red or green grapes
16 fat	48 walnut halves

Instructions

1 Preheat the oven to 350°F. Mist a 9 x 5-inch loaf pan with olive oil spray.

2 Combine the eggs, beans, spices, and tamari in a food processor or blender. Cover and blend until smooth. Pour into a 2-quart mixing bowl. Add the ground beef, oats, onion, bell pepper, celery, garlic powder, and ½ cup of the tomato sauce. Mix with clean bare hands and press into the loaf pan. Top with the remaining ½ cup tomato sauce.

3 Bake uncovered for 1 to 1¼ hours, or until the meatloaf is firm to the touch and pulls away from the sides of the pan, and an instant read thermometer registers 160°F.

4 Bring the filtered water to boil in a 1½-quart saucepan. Add the vegetables, cover, return to a boil, reduce the heat, and simmer 8 to 10 minutes or until tender, stirring occasionally. Drain the vegetables and sprinkle with the chives and cheese. Cover for 2 to 3 minutes, then transfer to 4 serving plates.

5 Cut the loaf into 8 slices. Place 2 slices on each of the 4 serving plates and serve immediately.

6 Toss the grapes with the walnuts and serve for dessert.

Tex-Mex Bean and Meat Loaf with Salad and Guacamole

Rachel Albert-Matesz

Prep: 20 minutes   **Yield:**   4 (4-block) servings
Cooking: 60 to 75 minutes

A well-stocked refrigerator, freezer, and pantry will make assembling this meal a breeze. If you prefer poultry, replace the ground meat with lean ground turkey, preferably breast meat.

Block Size	Ingredients
Bean and Meat Loaf	
2 protein	2 whole eggs **or** 4 egg whites
3 carbohydrate	¾ cup cooked kidney **or** black beans, drained
	1 tablespoon chili powder blend
	1 teaspoon ground cumin
	¼ teaspoon ground red pepper (optional)
	1 tablespoon tamari soy sauce (optional)
2 carbohydrate	⅓ cup non-instant rolled oats, uncooked
10 protein	15 ounces lean ground beef
2 carbohydrate	2 tablespoons dried onion flakes
2 carbohydrate	½ cup fresh or thawed frozen corn
½ carbohydrate	1 cup minced yellow or red bell pepper
2 carbohydrate	1 cup no-salt diced tomato with jalapeño, pureed and divided
Salad	
⅔ carbohydrate	7 cups romaine lettuce
1⅓ carbohydrate	1⅓ cups shredded carrot
1 carbohydrate	2 cups thinly sliced celery
½ carbohydrate	2 cups peeled, thinly sliced cucumber

4 protein	4 ounces grated, low-fat cheddar **or** Monterey Jack cheese (1 cup)

Guacamole

16 fat	1 cup chopped avocado
1 carbohydrate	Juice of 1 lime (about ⅓ cup)
	1 teaspoon hot sauce, or to taste
	Black pepper to taste

Instructions

1 Preheat the oven to 350°F. Mist a 9 x 5-inch loaf pan with olive oil spray.

2 Combine the eggs, beans, spices, and tamari in a food processor or blender. Cover, blend until smooth, and pour into a 2-quart mixing bowl. Add the oats, meat, onion, corn, bell pepper, and ½ cup of the tomato puree. Mix with clean bare hands and press into the pan. Top with the remaining ½ cup tomato sauce.

3 Bake uncovered for 1 to 1¼ hours, or until the meat loaf is firm to the touch and pulls away from sides of pan and an instant-read thermometer registers 160°F for beef (180°F for turkey).

4 Arrange the salad ingredients on 4 serving plates. In a small bowl, mash or beat the avocado, lime juice, hot sauce, and pepper until smooth. Spoon over the salads.

5 Cut the meat loaf into 8 slices. Place 2 slices on each of the 4 serving plates and serve immediately.

Glorious Garlic and Onion Dip and Dressing

Rachel Albert-Matesz

Prep: 15 minutes

Yield: 3 heaping cups; 9 servings
(⅓ cup = 4 fat blocks)

This dressing is great on green and main-dish salads or as a dip for raw or steamed chilled veggies. Each serving contains only ⅓ of a protein block and ⅓ of a carb block, which you don't have to count.

Block Size	Ingredients
3 protein, 3 carbohydrate	1½ cups organic low-fat yogurt, such as Stonyfield Farms
37 fat	1 cup Nayonnaise (soy-based sandwich spread)
	1 tablespoon minced fresh **or** 1 teaspoon dried chives
	1 tablespoon minced fresh **or** 1 teaspoon dried parsley
	⅛ teaspoon ground black pepper
	¼ teaspoon finely ground sea salt, or to taste

Instructions

Combine all the ingredients in a bowl. Stir or whisk until blended, cover, and refrigerate. Use within 2 weeks.

Three-Onion Dip and Dressing

Rachel Albert-Matesz

Prep: 10 minutes   **Yield:**   3 heaping cups; 9 servings
                                              (⅓ cup = 4 fat blocks)

Here's a reduced-fat version of a popular dip that doubles as a salad dressing. Try it over tossed green salads and shredded cabbage salad (for coleslaw), or use it to dunk raw veggie sticks or steamed and chilled broccoli, cauliflower, green beans, or asparagus spears. Each serving contains only ⅓ of a protein block and ⅓ of a carb block, which you don't have to count.

Block Size	Ingredients
3 protein, 3 carbohydrate	1½ cups organic low-fat yogurt, such as Stonyfield Farms
37 fat	1 cup Nayonnaise (soy-based sandwich spread)
	½ cup finely minced celery ribs or tops
	2 tablespoons minced fresh **or** 2 teaspoons dried chives
	2 tablespoons minced fresh onion
	2 teaspoons onion powder
	2 tablespoons minced fresh **or** 2 teaspoons dried parsley
	¼ teaspoon ground white pepper
	¼ teaspoon finely ground sea salt, or to taste

Instructions

Combine all ingredients in a bowl. Stir or whisk until blended, then cover and refrigerate. Use within 2 weeks.

Herb Garden Dip and Dressing

Rachel Albert-Matesz

Prep: 15 minutes

Yield: 3 heaping cups ; 9 servings
(⅓ cup = 4 fat blocks)

Use this to top green or main-dish salads, or as a dip for raw or steamed, chilled veggies. Each serving contains only ⅓ of a protein block and ⅓ of a carb block, which you don't have to count.

Block Size	Ingredients
37 fat	1 cup Nayonnaise (soy-based sandwich spread)
	1 tablespoon minced fresh **or** 1 teaspoon dried chives
	1 tablespoon minced fresh **or** 1 teaspoon dried parsley
	1 tablespoon minced fresh **or** 1 teaspoon dried tarragon
	2 teaspoons minced fresh **or** ⅔ teaspoon dried basil
	1 teaspoon minced fresh **or** ⅓ teaspoon dried oregano
3 protein, 3 carbohydrate	1½ cups organic low-fat yogurt, such as Stonyfield Farms
	¼ cup minced scallions **or** sweet white onion
	⅓ teaspoon ground white pepper
	¼ teaspoon finely ground sea salt, or to taste

Instructions

If you're using dried herbs, crumble them into a medium bowl. Add the rest of the ingredients and stir or whisk until blended. Cover and refrigerate. Use within 2 weeks.

Russian Yogurt Dip and Dressing

Rachel Albert-Matesz

Prep: 15 minutes   **Yield:**   2½ heaping cups; 5 servings
                                                     (½ cup = 4 fat blocks)

Here's a terrific dip for raw or steamed chilled veggies, and chicken breast strips or fish.
Try it as a dressing for green or main-dish salads.

Block Size	Ingredients
2 protein, 2 carbohydrate	1 cup organic low-fat yogurt, such as Stonyfield Farm
20 fat	½ cup Nayonnaise (soy-based sandwich spread)
3 carbohydrate	¼ cup plus 2 tablespoons fruit-sweetened ketchup
	2 tablespoons grated fresh **or** bottled horseradish
	3 tablespoons minced fresh parsley
	1½ teaspoon Worcestershire sauce (regular or vegetarian)
	2 tablespoons grated onion
	⅛ teaspoon ground black pepper
	¼ teaspoon finely ground sea salt, or to taste

Instructions

Combine all the ingredients in a bowl. Stir or whisk until blended, then cover and
refrigerate. Use within 2 weeks.

Yogurt Dill Dip and Dressing

Rachel Albert-Matesz

Prep: 15 minutes

Yield: 3 heaping cups; 9 servings
(⅓ cup = 4 fat blocks)

This makes a great dip for steamed and chilled broccoli and cauliflower, raw carrot and celery sticks, and grilled chicken breast strips. You can also serve it over green and main dish salads that include fish or chicken. Each serving contains only ⅓ of a protein block and ⅓ of a carb block, which you don't have to count. If you love mustard, add some.

Block Size	Ingredients
3 protein, 3 carbohydrate	1½ cups organic low-fat yogurt, such as Stonyfield Farms
37 fat	1 cup Nayonnaise (soy-based sandwich spread)
	¼ cup minced fresh **or** 1 tablespoon dried dill
	¼ cup minced celery
	¼ teaspoon ground white or black pepper
	1 teaspoon garlic powder (optional)
	¼ cup drained capers **or** sea salt to taste (optional)

Instructions

Combine all the ingredients in a bowl. Stir or whisk until blended, then cover and refrigerate. Use within 2 weeks.

Yogurt Ranch Dip and Dressing

Rachel Albert-Matesz

Prep: 15 minutes

Yield: 2 heaping cups; 8 servings
(¼ cup = 4 fat blocks)

Use this to top green and main-dish salads or as a dip for raw or steamed chilled veggies. Each serving contains only ⅛ of a protein block and ⅛ of a carb block, which you don't have to count.

Block Size	Ingredients
1 protein, 1 carbohydrate	1 cup cultured buttermilk
1 carbohydrate	Juice of 1 lime (2½ to 3 tablespoons)
37 fat	1 cup Nayonnaise (soy-based sandwich spread)
	1½ tablespoons minced fresh **or** 1½ teaspoons dried chives
	1½ tablespoons minced fresh **or** 1½ teaspoons dried parsley
	2 tablespoons minced scallions (green onions)
	1 medium garlic clove, pressed, **or** ⅛ teaspoon garlic powder, or to taste
	¼ teaspoon ground white pepper
	¼ teaspoon finely ground sea salt, or to taste

Instructions

Combine all the ingredients in a bowl. Stir or whisk until blended, then cover and refrigerate. Use within 2 weeks.

Yogurt Thousand Island Dip and Dressing

Rachel Albert-Matesz

Prep: 15 minutes

Yield: 3 heaping cups; 6 servings
(½ cup = 4 fat blocks)

Use this as a dip for raw or steamed chilled veggies and chicken breast strips or fish, or try it over tossed green or main-dish salads.

Block Size	Ingredients
2 protein, 2 carbohydrate	1 cup organic low-fat yogurt, such as Stonyfield Farms
23 fat	⅔ cup Nayonnaise (soy-based sandwich spread)
3 carbohydrate	¼ cup plus 2 tablespoons fruit-sweetened ketchup
	¼ cup Cascadian Farms natural dill relish
	1 tablespoon minced fresh chives
	2 tablespoons minced fresh parsley
	¾ teaspoon dried basil, crumbled
	⅛ teaspoon ground white or black pepper

Instructions

Combine all the ingredients in a bowl. Stir or whisk until blended, then cover and refrigerate. Use within 2 weeks.

Reduced-Fat Apricot-Mustard Dressing

Rachel Albert-Matesz

Prep: 5 minutes
Cooking: 10 to 15 minutes

Yield: 2 cups; 8 servings
(¼ cup = 4 fat blocks)

This sweet, creamy, and slightly spicy dressing makes a wonderful topping for tossed green salads that contain fresh fruit, chicken, turkey, seafood, or lean meat.

Block Size	Ingredients
	1 cup filtered water
8 carbohydrate	½ cup fruit-sweetened apricot jam
	2 teaspoons garlic powder **or** 4 small garlic cloves, pressed
	1 tablespoon Dijon mustard
	¼ teaspoon finely ground sea salt
32 fat	3 tablespoons plus 1⅔ teaspoons sesame oil
1 carbohydrate	4 teaspoons arrowroot starch
	1 teaspoon apple fiber powder **or** ¼ teaspoon guar gum **or** xanthan gum (optional but desirable)
	⅛ teaspoon ground black pepper
	¼ cup brown rice vinegar **or** red wine vinegar

Instructions

1 Combine and puree all the ingredients except the vinegar in a blender or food processor. Pour into a small saucepan and bring to a low boil over medium heat. Reduce the heat to medium low and simmer until clear, syrupy, and thick, stirring constantly, about 10 minutes. Whisk in the vinegar and pour into a glass jar.

2 Cool the dressing at room temperature; it will thicken more as it cools. Cover and refrigerate. Use within 1 week.

Reduced-Fat Raspberry Dressing

Rachel Albert-Matesz

Prep: 5 minutes   **Yield:**   2 cups; 8 servings
Cooking: 10 to 15 minutes   (¼ cup = 4 fat blocks)

Try this dressing over salads with mesclun, baby greens, or spring greens. If the salad contains fresh berries, orange or tangerine slices, sliced pears, pork loin, salmon, chicken, or duck breast, all the better!

Block Size	Ingredients
	1 cup filtered water
8 carbohydrate	½ cup fruit-sweetened raspberry jam
	1 tablespoon Dijon mustard
	¼ teaspoon finely ground sea salt
32 fat	3 tablespoons plus 1⅔ teaspoons sesame oil
1 carbohydrate	4 teaspoons arrowroot starch
	1 teaspoon apple fiber powder **or** ¼ teaspoon guar gum or xanthan gum
	⅛ teaspoon ground white pepper
	¼ cup brown rice vinegar **or** red wine vinegar

Instructions

1 Combine and puree all the ingredients except the vinegar in a blender or food processor. Pour into a small saucepan and bring to a low boil over medium heat. Reduce the heat to medium low and simmer until clear, syrupy, and thick, stirring constantly, about 10 minutes. Whisk in the vinegar and pour into a glass jar.

2 Cool the dressing at room temperature; it will thicken more as it cools. Cover and refrigerate. Use within 1 week.

Snacks

Zone snacks have a very important role in the Zone dietary plan. They're not just a fun diversion to break up the day. Rather, they serve as hormonal touchups, taking us through the times when we don't have a meal for more than four to five hours. The first Zone snack is eaten either between breakfast and lunch or between lunch and dinner, depending upon which is the longer time span. For instance, a person who gets up at 6 A.M. should eat breakfast by 7. If that person doesn't eat lunch until 1 or 2 P.M., then a Zone snack should be eaten between breakfast and lunch. On the other hand, a person who eats breakfast at 9 A.M. will have less time between breakfast and lunch and more time between lunch and dinner, which means the snack should be eaten in the afternoon. The second Zone snack is eaten about one hour before bedtime to prevent nocturnal hypoglycemia.

A Zone snack is really a mini-Zone meal. Each contains 1 block of protein, 1 block of carbohydrate, and 1 block of fat. The following list of snack ideas come from various Zone books and www.drsears.com and also offers some new options for snacking in the Zone.

Zone snack sizes are the same for men and women.

Deviled Eggs with Hummus

2 hard-boiled eggs
¼ cup hummus (contains fat)
Paprika to taste

Slice the eggs in half, discard the yolks, and fill each egg white with 1 tablespoon hummus. Top with paprika to taste.

Low-Fat Cottage Cheese and Fruit

¼ cup low-fat cottage cheese
⅓ cup "lite" fruit cocktail **or** ½ cup pineapple **or** ½ cup blueberries **or**
    ½ chopped apple **or** ⅓ cup unsweetened applesauce **or** 1 block of your favorite
    Zone-favorable fruit
1 macadamia nut **or** 3 almonds

Tomato and Low-Fat Mozzarella Salad

2 tomatoes, diced or sliced
⅓ teaspoon extra-virgin olive oil
Balsamic vinegar to taste
1 garlic clove, minced
1 ounce skim mozzarella cheese, grated
1 teaspoon chopped fresh basil leaves

Place the tomatoes on a plate. In a small bowl, whisk together the olive oil, vinegar, and garlic. Pour the dressing over the tomatoes. Top with the cheese and basil.

Tuna with Hummus

1 ounce canned tuna packed in water
¼ cup hummus

Drain the tuna fish and mix with the hummus.

Cottage Cheese and Salsa

¼ cup low-fat cottage cheese
½ cup salsa
1 tablespoon guacamole

Mix the ingredients in a small bowl.

Waldorf Salad

1 cup sliced celery
¼ apple, diced
1 teaspoon "light" mayonnaise
1 pecan, crushed
1 ounce part-skim **or** "soft" cheese

Mix the celery, apple, and mayonnaise in a small bowl. Sprinkle the pecan pieces on top. Serve the cheese on the side.

Low-Fat Yogurt and Nuts

½ cup plain low-fat yogurt
1 teaspoon slivered almonds or 1 macadamia nut

Spinach Salad

1 spinach side salad
2 hard-boiled egg whites, sliced
⅛ cup Mandarin oranges, canned in water
⅛ teaspoon olive oil
Balsamic vinegar to taste

Place the spinach on a plate. Top with egg whites and oranges. Whisk together the olive oil and vinegar and pour over the salad.

Veggies and Dip

2 ounces firm tofu
⅛ teaspoon olive oil
Dry onion soup mix to taste
1 cup celery sticks
1 green pepper, sliced

In a small bowl, blend the tofu, olive oil, and soup mix. Serve with the veggies.

Tomatoes and Low-Fat Cottage Cheese

2 tomatoes, sliced
¼ cup low-fat cottage cheese
6 peanuts

Place the tomato slices on a plate. Top with the cottage cheese and peanuts.

Chef Salad

1 lettuce side salad
1 ounce sliced turkey or ham
¼ cup kidney beans
⅛ teaspoon olive oil
Balsamic vinegar to taste

Place the lettuce in a bowl. Add the turkey or ham and kidney beans and toss with the olive oil and vinegar.

Ham and Fruit

4 slices Hillshire Farms 97 percent fat-free deli ham
½ apple
1 macadamia nut

Applesauce and Low-Fat Cheese

⅓ cup unsweetened applesauce

1 teaspoons slivered almonds

1 ounce low-fat cheese

Top the applesauce with the almonds and serve the cheese on the side.

Berries and Low-Fat Cheese

½ cup blueberries **or** 1 cup strawberries

1 ounce low-fat mozzarella cheese

6 peanuts

Wine and Cheese

4 ounces red **or** white wine

1 ounce cheese

The following snacks are popular with kids:

Cheese and Apple

½ teaspoon natural peanut butter

½ apple

1 ounce part-skim mozzarella string cheese

Spread the peanut butter on the apple and serve the cheese on the side.

Berry Smoothie

7 grams protein powder
1 cup frozen raspberries, defrosted
1 teaspoon slivered almonds

Blend the ingredients in a blender until smooth.

Taco Salad

1½ ounces ground turkey
Taco seasoning, to taste
1 lettuce side salad
1 tablespoon salsa
¼ cup black beans
1 tablespoon guacamole

Spray cooking spray into a small, nonstick sauté pan. Over medium heat, cook the turkey and sprinkle with taco seasoning. Place the lettuce on a plate and top with the turkey, salsa, beans, and guacamole.

CREATING YOUR OWN ZONE SNACKS

You can create an infinite variety of your very own Zone-favorable snacks. Pick and choose 1 protein, 1 carbohydrate, and 1 fat choice from the list below.

Protein Choices

¼ cup low-fat cottage cheese

1 ounce part-skim or "lite" mozzarella

2 ounces part-skim or "lite" ricotta cheese

1 ounce sliced turkey, ham, or chicken

1 ounce tuna packed in water

1 piece string cheese

1½ ounces deli meat

Carbohydrate Choices

½ apple

3 apricots

1 kiwi

1 tangerine

⅓ cup "lite" fruit cocktail

½ pear

1 cup strawberries

¾ cup blackberries

½ orange

½ cup grapes

8 cherries

½ nectarine

1 peach

1 plum

½ cup crushed pineapple

1 cup raspberries

½ cup blueberries

½ grapefruit

Fat Choices

3 green or black olives

1 macadamia nut

1 tablespoon avocado or guacamole

3 almonds

6 peanuts

2 pecans

½ teaspoon almond butter

½ teaspoon natural peanut butter

For other snack ideas, check out the following great recipes, including smoothies, puddings, muffins, and even frozen pops.

SNACK RECIPES

Blueberry-Peach and Yogurt Smoothie

Rachel Albert-Matesz

Prep: 10 minutes   **Yield:**   1 (4-block) meal or
                                                     4 (1-block) snacks

If you're preparing smoothies for two people for a meal, you can whip up a double batch at once. If you're serving more people, you'll have to make several batches.

Block Size	Ingredients
4 fat	8 unsalted cashews
1 protein, 1 carbohydrate	½ cups organic low-fat yogurt; ⅔ cup if yogurt does not contain nonfat dry milk
3 protein	1-ounce scoop vanilla egg white protein **or** whey protein powder
1 carbohydrate	1 cup frozen sliced peaches **or** 1 sliced fresh peach
2 carbohydrate	1 cup fresh blueberries **or** 1 cup frozen, unsweetened blueberries
	¼ teaspoon ground cinnamon **or** apple pie spice
	2 teaspoons apple fiber powder (optional)
	¼ cup filtered water **or** 2 ice cubes (optional)
	¹⁄₁₆ to ⅛ teaspoon stevia extract powder **or** 2 to 4 drops stevia extract liquid (optional)

Instructions

1 Pulverize the cashews in a blender. Add the yogurt, protein powder, peaches, blueberries, cinnamon or apple pie spice, and apple fiber, if desired. Cover and process until smooth, stopping to scrape down sides with spatula. Add ¼ cup water for a thinner texture or 2 ice cubes for a frostier texture. Add the stevia powder or liquid if the protein powder is unsweetened and/or a sweeter taste is desired. Blend and taste again.

2 Pour into 1 tall glass for a meal or 4 small cups for snacks and serve immediately. Or, pour into a wide-mouth thermos or thermoses and chill or freeze for later use. Allow a large frozen smoothie to thaw for several hours in the refrigerator or a cooler.

Variation

Blueberry-Peach and Yogurt Pops

Yield: 4 (1-block) snacks

Pour the blended mixture into 4 small paper cups or freezer pop molds. Freeze until firm. If using paper cups, place a stick into each cup after 1 to 2 hours, when mixture has started to ice up, then continue to freeze. Or, serve the mixture with spoons. Allow the cups to rest at room temperature for 10 minutes before serving, or run under warm water to loosen them from the molds.

Blueberry and Banana Cream Freeze

Rachel Albert-Matesz

Prep: 10 minutes

Yield: 1 (4-block) meal or
4 (1-block) snacks

Eat this as a soft serve or as frozen pops. Either way, it makes a tasty Zone snack or light meal.

Block Size	Ingredients
4 fat	¼ cup low-fat organic sour cream
	¼ cup filtered water
4 protein	1⅓ ounces vanilla egg white protein **or** whey protein
	¼ teaspoon ground cinnamon **or** apple pie spice
	1 teaspoon pure vanilla extract in a nonalcoholic base **or** ½ teaspoon pure vanilla in alcohol
1 carbohydrate	⅓ cup sliced frozen banana
3 carbohydrate	1½ cups frozen blueberries
	2 teaspoons apple fiber powder (optional)
	2 ice cubes
	1⁄16 teaspoon stevia extract powder **or** 2 to 3 drops stevia extract liquid (optional)

Instructions

1 Combine the sour cream, water, protein powder, cinnamon, vanilla, banana, and blueberries in a blender. Add the apple fiber if using. Cover and process until smooth, stopping to scrape down the sides with spatula. Add ice, one cube at a time, as needed to create a thick, frosty texture. Taste and add stevia if protein powder is unsweetened or a sweeter taste is desired. Blend and taste again, adjusting the sweetening as needed.

2 Pour and scrape into 1 tall glass for a meal or 4 cups for snacks and serve immediately. Or, pour into one or more wide-mouth thermos bottles and chill or freeze for later.

Variation

Blueberry and Banana Cream Pops

Yield: 4 (1-block) snacks

Pour the blended mixture into 4 small paper cups or freezer pop molds. Freeze until firm. If using paper cups, place a stick in each cup after 1 to 2 hours, when the mixture has started to ice up, then continue to freeze. Or, serve the mixture with spoons. Allow the cups to rest at room temperature for 10 minutes before serving, or run under warm water to loosen them from the molds.

Blueberry-Banana and Macadamia Nut Smoothie

Rachel Albert-Matesz

Prep: 10 minutes   **Yield:**   1 (4-block) meal or
                                                      4 (1-block) snacks

Bananas add a smooth texture to this smoothie.

Block Size	Ingredients
1 protein, 1 carbohydrate	½ cup organic low-fat yogurt; ⅔ cup if yogurt does not contain nonfat dry milk
4 fat	4 unsalted macadamia nuts **or** 2 teaspoons macadamia nut butter
3 protein	1-ounce scoop vanilla egg white protein **or** whey protein powder
2 carbohydrate	1 cup fresh blueberries **or** 1 cup frozen blueberries
1 carbohydrate	⅓ banana **or** ⅓ cup sliced frozen banana
	¼ teaspoon ground cinnamon **or** ⅛ teaspoon ground nutmeg
	2 teaspoons apple fiber powder (optional)
	1/16 to ⅛ teaspoon stevia extract powder or liquid (optional)
	¼ cup filtered water or 2 ice cubes (optional)

Instructions

1 Combine the yogurt, nuts or nut butter, protein powder, blueberries, banana, and cinnamon or nutmeg in a blender. Add the apple fiber powder if desired. Cover and process until smooth, stopping to scrape down the sides with spatula. Add stevia if the protein powder is unsweetened or a sweeter taste is desired. Blend and taste again.

2 Pour into 1 tall glass for a meal or 4 small cups for 4 snacks and serve immediately. Or, pour into a wide-mouth thermos or thermoses and chill or freeze for later, then transfer frozen smoothies to the refrigerator or a cooler and allow several hours for defrosting.

Variation

Blueberry-Banana and Macadamia Pops

Yield: 4 (1-block) snacks

Pour the blended mixture into 4 small paper cups or freezer pop molds. Freeze until firm. If using paper cups, place a stick in each cup after 1 to 2 hours, when mixture has started to ice up, then continue to freeze, or serve the mixture with spoons. Allow the cups to rest at room temperature for 10 minutes before serving or run under warm water to loosen them from the molds.

Cherry-Peach and Cashew Freeze

Rachel Albert-Matesz

Prep: 10 minutes

Yield: 1 (4-block) meal or
4 (1-block) snacks

The marriage of pitted, unsweetened "sweet" cherries and sliced frozen peaches makes a delicious breakfast or snack. You can eat it as a soft serve or as frozen pops.

Block Size	Ingredients
4 fat	8 cashews
	¼ cup filtered water
4 protein	1⅓ ounces vanilla egg white protein **or** whey protein
	⅛ teaspoon ground nutmeg
	⅛ teaspoon ground cinnamon
	1 teaspoon pure vanilla extract in a nonalcoholic base **or** ½ teaspoon pure vanilla in alcohol
1 carbohydrate	1 cup sliced frozen peaches
3 carbohydrate	¾ of a 12-ounce package frozen, pitted, unsweetened "sweet" cherries (such as Big Valley), about 1 cup
	2 teaspoons apple fiber powder (optional)
	2 ice cubes (optional)
	¹⁄₁₆ teaspoon stevia extract powder **or** 2 to 3 drops stevia extract liquid (optional)

Instructions

1 Combine the cashews, water, protein powder, nutmeg, cinnamon, vanilla, and fruit in blender. Add the apple fiber if desired. Cover and process until smooth, stopping to scrape down the sides with spatula. Add ice one cube at a time as needed to create a thick, frosty texture. Taste and add stevia if protein powder is unsweetened or a sweeter taste is desired. Blend and taste again, adjusting the sweetening as needed.

2 Pour and scrape into 1 tall glass for a meal or 4 cups for snacks and serve immediately. Or pour into one or more wide-mouth thermos bottles and chill or freeze for later.

Variation

Cherry-Peach and Cashew Pops

Yield: 4 (1-block) snacks

Pour the blended mixture into 4 small paper cups or freezer pop molds. Freeze until firm. If using paper cups, place a stick in each cup after 1 to 2 hours, when the mixture has started to ice up, then continue to freeze. Or serve the mixture with spoons. Allow the cups to rest at room temperature for 10 minutes before serving or run under warm water to loosen them from the molds.

Cocoa Berry Smoothie

Rachel Albert-Matesz

Prep: 10 minutes

Yield: 1 (4-block) meal or
4 (1-block) snacks

If your freezer is stocked with frozen fruit, a nourishing snack or breakfast will only be minutes away. Buy single fruits or fruit blends; just make sure they are unsweetened. Berries pack the most antioxidants for your carb blocks.

Block Size	Ingredients
	½ cup filtered water
4 fat	8 unsalted cashews **or** 2 teaspoons cashew butter
4 protein	1⅓ ounces vanilla egg white protein **or** whey protein
3 carbohydrate	1½ cups fresh blueberries **or** frozen blueberries (¾ of a 12-ounce bag)
1 carbohydrate	2 teaspoons fructose powder
	2 teaspoons unsweetened cocoa
	¼ teaspoon ground cinnamon
	2 teaspoons apple fiber powder (optional)
	1/16 to ⅛ teaspoon stevia extract powder or liquid (optional)
	2 to 3 ice cubes (optional)

Instructions

1 Combine all the ingredients except the stevia and ice in a blender. Cover and process until smooth, stopping to scrape down sides with a spatula. Add 1 ice cube at a time as needed to create a thick frosty texture. Add $\frac{1}{16}$ teaspoon stevia if protein powder is unsweetened and/or a sweeter taste is desired. Blend, taste, and adjust as needed.

2 Pour into 1 tall glass for a meal or 4 small cups for 4 snacks and serve immediately. Or pour into a wide-mouth thermos or thermoses and chill or freeze for later. Transfer the frozen smoothies to refrigerator or cooler and allow several hours for thawing.

Variation

Replace fructose with $\frac{1}{3}$ cup fresh or $\frac{1}{2}$ cup frozen mango. Add an additional $\frac{1}{16}$ teaspoon stevia if a sweeter taste is desired.

Strawberry-Mango-Pineapple Smoothie

Rachel Albert-Matesz

Prep: 10 minutes   **Yield:**   1 (4-block) meal or
                                                         4 (1-block) snacks

Most supermarkets sell frozen fruit blends. The pineapple-mango-strawberry blend makes fantastic smoothies for snacks, breakfast on the go, or a light and easy-to-assemble evening meal.

Block Size	Ingredients
1 protein, 1 carbohydrate	½ cup organic low-fat yogurt; ⅔ cup if yogurt does not contain nonfat dry milk
4 fat	8 unsalted cashews
3 protein	1 ounce scoop vanilla egg white protein **or** whey protein
1 carbohydrate	1 cup frozen **or** 1 cup fresh strawberries
1 carbohydrate	⅓ cup fresh **or** ½ cup frozen cubed mango
1 carbohydrate	½ cup frozen **or** ½ cup fresh pineapple slices
	1 teaspoon minced fresh or bottled ginger root **or** ¼ teaspoon ground ginger
	2 teaspoons apple fiber powder (optional)
	¼ cup filtered water or 2 ice cubes (optional)
	⅟₁₆ to ⅛ teaspoon stevia extract powder or liquid (optional)

Instructions

1 Add the yogurt, cashews, protein powder, strawberries, mango, pineapple, and ginger to a blender. Add the apple fiber if desired. Cover and process until smooth, stopping to scrape down the sides with spatula. Add ¼ cup cold water for a thinner texture or 2 ice cubes frostier texture. Add ⅟₁₆ teaspoon stevia if the protein powder is unsweetened or a sweeter taste is desired. Blend and taste.

2 Pour into 1 tall glass for a meal or 4 small cups for 4 snacks and serve immediately. Or pour into one or more wide-mouth thermos bottles and chill or freeze for later. Transfer the frozen smoothies to the refrigerator or cooler and allow several hours for defrosting.

Variation

Strawberry-Mango-Pineapple Pops

Yield: 4 (1-block) snacks

Pour the blended mixture into 4 small paper cups or freezer pop molds. Freeze until firm. If using paper cups, place a stick in each cup after 1 to 2 hours, when the mixture has started to ice up, then continue to freeze. Or serve the mixture with spoons. Allow the cups to rest at room temperature for 10 minutes before serving or run under warm water to loosen them from the mold.

Melon, Cherry, Grape, and Yogurt Smoothie

Rachel Albert-Matesz

Prep: 10 minutes

Yield: 1 (4-block) meal or
4 (1-block) snacks

Look for a frozen melon, cherry, and grape blend in your supermarket's freezer section or slice and freeze fresh fruit at home, making it ready for a later date. Whip up a double recipe for breakfast for two, or make extra portions to freeze in paper cups for snacks.

Block Size	Ingredients
1 protein, 1 carbohydrate	½ cup organic low-fat yogurt (⅔ cup if yogurt does not contain nonfat dry milk)
4 fat	2 teaspoons unsalted, unsweetened almond butter
3 protein	1-ounce scoop vanilla egg white protein **or** vanilla whey protein
1 carbohydrate	¾ cup sliced fresh honeydew, cantaloupe, or Crenshaw melon **or** 1 cup frozen melon balls
1 carbohydrate	½ cup seedless red grapes **or** ½ cup frozen grapes
1 carbohydrate	⅓ cup fresh, pitted unsweetened "sweet" cherries **or** ½ cup frozen unsweetened "sweet" cherries (not thawed)
	¼ teaspoon dried ginger **or** 1 teaspoon minced fresh or bottled ginger root
	2 teaspoons apple fiber powder (optional)
	¼ cup filtered water **or** 2 ice cubes (optional)
	¹⁄₁₆ to ⅛ teaspoon stevia extract powder **or** 2 to 4 drops stevia liquid (optional)

Instructions

1 Combine the yogurt, nut butter, protein powder, melon, grapes, cherries, and ginger. Add the apple fiber if desired. Cover and process until smooth, stopping to scrape down the sides with spatula. Add ¼ cup water for a thinner texture or 2 ice cubes for a frostier texture. Add ⅟₁₆ teaspoon stevia if protein powder is unsweetened or a sweeter taste is desired. Blend and taste again.

2 Pour into 1 tall glass for a meal or 4 small cups for snacks and serve immediately. Or pour into a wide-mouth thermos or thermoses and chill or freeze for later use. Allow a large frozen smoothie to thaw for several hours in the refrigerator or a cooler.

Variation

Melon, Cherry, Grape, and Yogurt Pops

Yields   4 (1-block) snacks

Pour the blended mixture into 4 small paper cups or freezer pop molds. Freeze until firm. If using paper cups, place a stick in each cup after 1 to 2 hours, once the mixture has started to ice up, then continue to freeze. Allow the cups to rest at room temperature for 10 minutes before serving or run under warm water to loosen them from the molds.

Very Cherry Yogurt Smoothie

Rachel Albert-Matesz

Prep: 10 minutes

Yield: 1 (4-block) meal or
4 (1-block) snacks

Stock up on frozen pitted, unsweetened "sweet" cherries. They'll enhance your yogurt and your morning.

Block Size	Ingredients
1 protein, 1 carbohydrate	½ cups organic low-fat yogurt; ⅔ cup if yogurt does not contain nonfat dry milk
4 fat	8 unsalted cashews
3 protein	1-ounce scoop vanilla egg white protein **or** whey protein
3 carbohydrate	¾ of a 12-ounce package frozen pitted, unsweetened "sweet" cherries (such as Big Valley) **or** 1 cup pitted, sweet cherries
	1 teaspoon minced fresh or bottled ginger **or** ¼ teaspoon dried ginger
	2 teaspoons apple fiber powder (optional)
	¼ cup filtered water **or** 2 ice cubes (optional)
	⅟₁₆ to ⅛ teaspoon stevia extract powder **or** 2 to 4 drops stevia extract liquid (optional)

Instructions

1 Combine the yogurt, cashews, protein powder, cherries, and ginger. Add the apple fiber if desired. Cover and process until smooth, stopping to scrape down sides with spatula. Add ¼ cup water for a thinner texture or 2 ice cubes for a frostier texture. Add ¹⁄₁₆ teaspoon stevia if the protein powder is unsweetened or a sweeter taste is desired. Blend and taste again.

2 Pour into 1 tall glass for a meal or 4 small cups for snacks. Serve immediately or pour into one or more wide-mouth thermos bottles and chill or freeze for later. Allow a large, frozen smoothie to thaw for several hours in the refrigerator or a cooler.

Variation

Very Cherry Yogurt Pops

Yield: 4 (1-block) snacks

Pour the blended mixture into 4 small paper cups or freezer pop molds. Freeze until firm. If using paper cups, place a stick in each cup after 1 to 2 hours, when the mixture has started to ice up, then continue to freeze or serve the mixture with spoons. Allow the cups to rest at room temperature for 10 minutes before serving or run under warm water to loosen them from the molds.

Frozen Blueberry Yogurt

www.drsears.com

Prep: 5 minutes

Yield: 1 (3-block) meal or
3 (1-block) snacks

Block Size	Ingredients
1 protein,1 carbohydrate	½ cup organic low-fat yogurt; ⅔ cup if yogurt does not contain nonfat dry milk
2 carbohydrates	1 cup frozen blueberries
2 protein	½ cup cottage cheese
3 fat	1 tablespoon slivered almonds
1 carbohydrate	2 teaspoons fructose powder

Instructions

Place all the ingredients in a blender or food processor and blend until smooth.

Watermelon-Berry Cooler

Rachel Albert-Matesz

Prep: 10 minutes

Yield: 1 (4-block) meal or
4 (1-block) snacks

If you don't want to mess with removing watermelon seeds, look for seedless watermelon. If you're serving this as a breakfast for more than one person, you'll have to make several batches.

Block Size	Ingredients
1 protein, 1 carbohydrate	½ cup organic low-fat yogurt; ⅔ cup if yogurt does not contain nonfat dry milk
4 fat	8 cashews
3 protein	1-ounce scoop vanilla egg white protein **or** whey protein powder
2 carbohydrate	1½ cups fresh or frozen sliced seedless **or** seeded watermelon
1 carbohydrate	½ cup fresh **or** ½ cup frozen blueberries, thawed
	1 teaspoon peeled, minced fresh ginger **or** bottled ginger juice
	¼ cup filtered water **or** 2 ice cubes (optional)
	1⁄16 to ⅛ teaspoon stevia extract powder **or** 2 to 4 drops stevia extract liquid (optional)

Instructions

1 Combine the yogurt, cashews, protein powder, watermelon, blueberries, and ginger in a blender. Cover and process until smooth, stopping to scrape down sides with a spatula. Add ¼ cup water for a thinner texture or 2 ice cubes for a frostier texture. Add ¹⁄₁₆ teaspoon stevia if the protein powder is unsweetened or a sweeter taste is desired. Blend and taste again.

2 Pour into 1 tall glass for a meal or 4 small cups for snacks and serve immediately. Or pour into a wide-mouth thermos or thermoses and chill or freeze for later use. Allow a large frozen smoothie to thaw for several hours in the refrigerator or a cooler.

Zoned Apple Pie Pudding

Rachel Albert-Matesz

Prep: 20 minutes   **Yield:** 4 (1-block) snacks
Cooking: 2 to 3 minutes

This cross between apple pie and applesauce makes a great snack. If you don't have almond or cashew butter in the house, try it with peanut butter or substitute eight raw or toasted cashews.

Block Size	Ingredients
	¾ cup cold water
1 protein	1 tablespoon unflavored gelatin
4 fat	2 teaspoons unsweetened, unsalted almond butter **or** cashew butter
3 carbohydrate	1½ small sweet or tart-sweet apples (Fuji, Braeburn, JonaGold, Gala, Granny Smith, Macintosh, Pink Lady, Ginger Gold, or Cortland), cored, peeled if desired or waxed, halved, and diced
3 protein	1-ounce scoop vanilla whey protein **or** egg white protein powder
1 carbohydrate	2 teaspoons fructose powder
	½ teaspoon pure vanilla extract, preferably nonalcoholic
	½ teaspoon apple pie spice **or** ground cinnamon
	¼ cup ice water (optional)
	⅛ teaspoon stevia extract powder **or** liquid (optional)

Instructions

1 In a small saucepan, add the cold water and slowly sprinkle with gelatin. Warm the mixture over low heat until it is dissolved, 1 to 3 minutes. Pour the mixture into a blender or food processor; cover, and blend on low, then high, until frothy.

2 Add the almond or cashew butter, apples, protein powder, fructose powder, vanilla, and apple pie spice or cinnamon. Cover and blend until smooth, stopping to scrape down the sides with spatula. Add the ice water as needed to yield 2 cups of pudding, as measured on the side of the blender. Blend, taste, and adjust the sweetness with stevia if desired, and blend again.

3 Pour into 4 small serving dishes and chill until set. Use within 5 days.

Zoned Chocolate Pudding

Rachel Albert-Matesz

Prep: 20 minutes   **Cooking:** 2 to 3 minutes
Soaking: 30 minutes   **Yield:**   4 (1-block) snacks

Have your chocolate and eat it too—without going out of the Zone! Unlike most puddings, this one requires no messy mixing and cooking on top of the stove. Unflavored gelatin and a blender do all the work. Almond butter adds heart-healthy monounsaturated fats, and dates and fructose do the sweetening.

Block Size	Ingredients
	½ cup cold water
1 protein	1 tablespoon unflavored gelatin
4 fat	12 lightly toasted almonds **or** 2 teaspoons unsweetened, unsalted almond butter
3 carbohydrate	6 pitted dates
	2 teaspoons apple fiber powder
	1 tablespoon unsweetened cocoa
3 protein	1 ounce scoop vanilla whey protein **or** egg white protein powder
1 carbohydrate	2 teaspoons fructose powder
	1 teaspoon pure vanilla extract, preferably nonalcoholic
	½ teaspoon ground cinnamon
	¼ cup ice water
	⅛ to ¼ teaspoon stevia extract powder **or** liquid (optional)

Instructions

1 Add the cold water to a small saucepan and slowly sprinkle with gelatin. Warm the mixture over low heat until it is dissolved, 1 to 3 minutes. Add the almonds or almond butter and dates and soak for 30 minutes to soften. Pour the mixture into a blender or food processor; cover, and blend on low, then high, until smooth and creamy.

2 Add the apple fiber powder, cocoa, protein powder, fructose, vanilla, and cinnamon. Cover and blend until smooth, stopping to scrape down the sides with spatula. Add ice water and blend. Taste and adjust sweetness with stevia if a sweeter taste is desired, then blend again.

3 Pour into 4 small serving dishes and chill until set. Use within 5 days.

Variation

Zoned Chocolate Pudding Pops

In step 3, pour the mixture into 4 small paper cups. After ½ hour, insert a craft stick into each cup. Freeze until set. Peel off the paper to eat. Or, freeze the pudding in cups, allow to soften on the counter for 10 to 15 minutes, and eat with a spoon.

Zoned Chocolate Protein Prune Pudding

Rachel Albert-Matesz

Prep: 20 minutes
Soaking: 30 minutes

Cooking: 2 to 3 minutes
Yield: 4 (1-block) snacks

Both prunes and cocoa are rich in antioxidants. This recipe combines them with heart-healthy fats and protein to produce a delicious blood sugar-balancing snack.

Block Size	Ingredients
	¾ cup cold water
⅔ protein	2 teaspoons unflavored gelatin
2 carbohydrate	4 pitted prunes
4 fat	12 lightly toasted almonds **or** 2 teaspoons unsweetened, unsalted almond butter
	2 teaspoons apple fiber powder
	1½ tablespoons unsweetened cocoa
3⅓ protein	1⅓ ounce vanilla whey protein or egg white protein powder
2 carbohydrate	4 teaspoons fructose powder **or** 1 tablespoon agavé nectar
	1 teaspoon pure vanilla extract, preferably nonalcoholic
	¼ teaspoon ground cinnamon
	¼ cup ice water
	⅛ to ¼ teaspoon stevia extract powder **or** liquid (optional)

Instructions

1 Add the cold water to a small saucepan and slowly sprinkle with gelatin. Warm the mixture over low heat until it is dissolved, 1 to 3 minutes. Add the prunes and nuts or nut butter and soak for 30 minutes to soften. Pour the mixture into a blender or food processor, cover, and blend on low, then high, until smooth and creamy.

2 Add the apple fiber powder, cocoa, protein powder, fructose, vanilla, and cinnamon. Cover and blend until smooth, stopping to scrape down the sides with a spatula. Add the ice water, blend, add stevia if a sweeter taste is desired, and blend again.

3 Pour into 4 small serving dishes and chill until set. Use within 5 days.

Variation

Zoned Chocolate Prune Pudding Pops

In step 3, pour the mixture into 4 small paper cups. After ½ hour, insert a craft stick into each cup. Freeze until set. Peel off the paper to eat. Or, freeze the pudding in cups, allow to soften on the counter for 10 to 15 minutes, and eat with a spoon.

7

The Kids' Zone

> Our daughters were born in 1978 and 1980, long before Barry began his search for a diet in which food would be our best medicine. In those early days, I was clueless about nutrition. When my girls were small, I thought nothing was wrong with fixing the kids macaroni and cheese for dinner. Lunch bags were stuffed with sandwiches, potato chips, cookies, and an apple. Most of the time the apple came back to me at the end of the day. Imagine that.
>
> —*Lynn Sears*

Kids can be incredibly picky eaters. The story about our younger daughter in the Introduction is true—at one point she would only eat chicken for her protein choice and green apples and grapes for her carbohydrate choices. She often ate a grilled chicken Caesar salad on green lettuce and green grapes or a green Granny Smith apple for dinner. That was a bit monotonous, but at least it kept her in the Zone. Meal preparation couldn't have been simpler. We would get skinless, cooked chicken breast from the supermarket's deli and throw it in the microwave to heat it slightly. While it was warming, we opened an individual-size Caesar salad package from the grocery store and tossed it with the dressing provided, or our own healthier olive oil and vinegar recipe. We cut the chicken up and put it on top, and just to keep it interesting, put about four of the package's croutons on top of the salad greens and threw the rest away. Then out came the bowl of green grapes or green sliced apples, and that was that.

Until our daughter entered her late teens, she was a picky eater. Then all of a sudden she began to enjoy eating everything, including vegetables and fruits of all colors.

By the time the Zone concept entered our household, our older daughter was ten and our younger daughter was eight. As we began to bring our children into the Zone, we found that it was easier to regulate their consumption of proteins, carbohydrates, and fats by putting a lot of different bowls of carbohydrates on the table. In other words, don't put all your carbs in one basket. That way we could eyeball what our kids were eating.

The protein was easy to measure. We would put the correct amount on their plate, say two or three ounces of chicken. If they didn't eat it all, we knew they would eat a piece of string cheese.

Carbohydrates we put on the table included the proverbial bowl of grapes, a bowl of chickpeas or kidney beans for salads, and hummus on a small wedge of pita bread. Hummus also tastes great on a salad. If you use it as a dressing, eliminate any other fat because hummus contains both carbohydrates and fat. When you serve your children fruit, cut it up. A child will more readily eat an orange that's been peeled and sectioned or an apple that is seeded and cut in wedges.

Usually, a child of elementary school age eats 2-block meals, and a middle school or high school student graduates to 3 or more. Of course, each child is different. Some kids are still tiny in sixth grade, while others are much earlier bloomers. Take a cue from your children. If they are in the Zone, they will be eating the size portions that are right for them. The earlier children enter the Zone, the earlier it will become second nature for them to stay in the Zone. We've had numerous Zoner parents tell us that when somebody gives their child an apple, he or she asks for protein to go along with it. By the time they're teenagers, kids will be so used to the extra energy and mental acuity the Zone brings that they won't be as tempted to eat badly when they go out with their friends for dinner or lunch. If you must take them to a fast-food restaurant, follow the guidelines in chapter 4.

In a study conducted at Harvard Medical School in 1999 (*Pediatrics* 103: E26 1999), twelve obese teenage boys were given low glycemic-load and high glycemic-load meals containing the same number of calories. In essence, some of the boys were given a Zone meal and the others a meal based on the USDA Food Pyramid, which relies heavily on grains and starches. Both meals had the same number of calories. At the next meal the boys who had eaten the Zone meal consumed 25 percent fewer calories. Therein lies the power of the Zone dietary program. If you aren't as hungry, you don't eat as much food at the next meal.

Let's begin to bring your kids into the Zone. The Zone Food Block Guide on page 365 gives countless combinations to use to make Zone meals. Here are a few choices to get you started.

First come the protein choices pre-adolescent children should have at every meal.

Children should eat any combination of two of the following protein blocks at each meal. Each choice equals one block.

1 ounce lean beef **or** Canadian bacon **or** skinless chicken breast **or** canned tuna in water **or** low-fat cheese

1 egg **or** 1 piece string cheese **or** soy sausage link **or** soy hot dog (check the label)

1½ ounces ground turkey **or** lean ground beef **or** crabmeat **or** lobster **or** scallops **or** shrimp **or** deli meat

2 egg whites

3 strips turkey bacon

¼ cup cottage cheese or egg substitute

½ soy hamburger (check the label)

2 ounces firm tofu

Next add the carbohydrate choices.

Children should eat any combination of two of the following protein blocks at each meal. Each choice equals one block.

⅛ cup dry pearl barley (check the label; 1 block is 9 grams)

¼ cup black beans **or** chickpeas **or** kidney beans **or** lentils

⅓ cup water chestnuts **or** unsweetened applesauce **or** Mandarin oranges canned in water **or** fruit cocktail canned in water **or** steel-cut oatmeal

½ cup tomato sauce **or** blueberries **or** boysenberries **or** grapes **or** peaches canned in water **or** cubed pineapple

½ apple **or** grapefruit **or** nectarine **or** orange **or** pear

1 cup artichoke hearts **or** tomato (canned and chopped) **or** raspberries **or** strawberries (chopped fine) **or** spaghetti squash

1 kiwi **or** 1 nectarine **or** 1 peach **or** 1 plum

1½ cups green or wax beans **or** chopped onions **or** snow peas **or** chopped fresh tomatoes

1½ cucumbers

2 cups whole boiled mushrooms **or** zucchini **or** bell peppers **or** sliced celery **or** cherry tomatoes

3 cups cooked broccoli

Bread/toast (not more than 9 grams)

Finally, add two blocks of fat.

Children should eat any combination of two of the following fat blocks at each meal.

Each choice equals one block.

⅓ teaspoon olive oil

½ teaspoon tahini **or** almond butter **or** natural peanut butter

1 teaspoon slivered almonds

1 teaspoon light mayonnaise

1 macadamia nut

1 tablespoon avocado **or** guacamole

3 olives **or** pistachios **or** almonds

6 peanuts

It should also be noted that 1 cup of 1-percent milk contains one block of protein, one block of carbohydrate, and one block of fat.

Putting It All Together

So here's what a child's day might look like.

Breakfast (eaten within 1 hour of waking):

- 1 ounce Canadian bacon sautéed in ⅔ teaspoon olive oil, 1 ounce low-fat cheese melted on ½ piece of toast, and ½ orange cut in sections

- Two egg whites scrambled or ½ cup egg substitute, cooked in ⅓ teaspoon olive oil, 1 cup 1-percent milk, 1 peach

- Half a Zone muffin (see pages 61–68) and 1 cup 1-percent milk

- 2 low-fat string cheeses, ½ cup of grapes, 1 piece of toast topped with 1 teaspoon of natural peanut butter

- ½ cup low-fat cottage cheese mixed with ⅓ cup unsweetened applesauce, ½ cup pineapple, and 2 teaspoons slivered almonds

We can't overemphasize how important it is for a child to have a Zone breakfast within an hour of waking. That lesson was driven home to us one morning when a client visited our Zone Center. It was a school holiday, and she brought her six-year-old son along for her appointment. To say that the boy misbehaved is an incredible understatement. His antics included ripping up papers on a desk and taking pencils out of their holders and hurling them across the room. His mother was aghast and told us that her son had never acted like that before. We asked what she had fed him for breakfast. She said that "as a special treat" she had taken him to a restaurant for breakfast where he had eaten pancakes topped with a sugary blueberry syrup. The realization hit her that the "special treat" wasn't very special after all.

Lunch

A good lunch for an elementary school child might consist of:

- 1 string cheese, 1 small carton of low-fat milk, ½ cup grapes, 6 peanuts

- 2 ounces tuna fish in water, drained, mixed with 2 teaspoons light mayonnaise, 1 piece of low-carbohydrate bread (10 grams or less), 1 plum

- 1½ ounces julienne deli ham and 1½ ounces julienne deli turkey, served on a small bed of lettuce with olive oil and vinegar dressing (⅔ teaspoon olive oil plus vinegar to taste), and 1 apple

- Half a Zone muffin (pages 61–68), 1 ounce cooked skinless chicken breast, and ½ an apple spread with 1 teaspoon natural peanut butter

Just as it is for an adult, the timing of a child's daytime snack depends upon how much time elapses between two meals. If a child eats breakfast at 7 or 8 A.M. and has lunch between 11 and 12, then he or she should wait and have a snack after school. If the lunch hour comes at 1 P.M. or later during the school year, ask the child's teacher to allow a midmorning snack. If a child is in a childcare program, make sure the afternoon snack is one made at home and not provided at the daycare facility. Have you ever noticed how children are bouncing off the walls when their parents pick them up every afternoon? That's because the traditional midafternoon snack at a daycare center is cookies and apple juice, all carbohydrates—and bad ones at that.

Most of the snacks Americans give to their kids are bound to raise their insulin levels sky high. In the last thirty years the obesity rate for children has tripled. This means they are on a fast track toward diabetes and heart disease. Excess insulin production is also associated with attention deficit disorder and asthma—two conditions that have also seen epidemic surges in the last thirty years.

Snack foods to eliminate or greatly curtail include dry cereals, sodas and sweetened fruit drinks, canned pasta, popcorn, potato chips, and sweets of any kind.

Kid-friendly snacks include:

- 1 string cheese and ½ cup of grapes
- 1 Zone mini-muffin (divide the batter among 16 muffin cups)
- 1 ounce cooked chicken and ½ apple spread with ½ teaspoon natural peanut butter
- 1 cup 1-percent milk

Dinner

A good dinner for a child of elementary school age might be:

- 2 ounces chicken, 1½ cups green beans with a nice sauce (see ideas below), a green salad topped with ¼ cup hummus, and ½ orange
- 3 ounces shrimp with a dipping sauce (see ideas below), a fruit salad of ½ cup grapes and ½ cup pineapple, and 6 almonds
- 1 Boca smoked soy sausage, 1 piece of bread (9 grams) spread with 1 teaspoon almond butter, and 1 peach

Remember to have simple substitutions on hand. For instance, if your child won't eat chickpeas, have a bowl of grapes ready. Also, keep a supply of string cheese in the refrigerator. If your child won't finish the chicken, one or two pieces of string cheese will make sure adequate protein is consumed.

Use sauces to make food more appealing to kids. Instructions are given on Campbell's Soup cans, such as cream of mushroom and cream of chicken, on how to make a tasty meal cooked in soup. Even children who say they hate vegetables will eat them in soups and stews.

Packaged Knorr sauce mixes, such as Béarnaise and Hollandaise, will also make vegetables taste great. Just use 2 tablespoons of olive oil instead of the recommended butter. Tofu mixed with dry onion soup mix is also a good dipping sauce for raw broccoli and celery. Just tell the kids they're eating snow-covered trees. It worked for me when my kids were growing up. Check out the other delicious dip and dressing recipes that start on page 166.

And don't forget a snack before your child goes to bed. A glass of 1 percent milk might hit the spot, and it also might cause the little tyke to go to sleep earlier.

We also want to talk about another dietary dilemma in our family, when our older daughter became a lacto-ovo vegetarian at the age of fourteen in 1992. It was a challenge. We could use eggs and cheese, but just about the only soy product available back then was tofu, which at first looked like a disgusting, slimy mass, but we got used to cooking with it pretty quickly. Today there are a number of good-tasting soy products at the supermarket. People have to get used to using the gram method of Zoning when figuring out soy product portions, which we explain in chapter 8, The Can-Do Zone.

8

The Can-Do Zone

We hope by now you are familiar with either the hand-eye method or Zone Food Blocks and are able to construct a variety of meals. But what happens when you just want to open a can of soup or put a frozen dinner in the microwave? That's where gram counting comes in. You just have to learn three numbers. It isn't hard at all.

$$1 \text{ protein block} = 7 \text{ grams}$$
$$1 \text{ carbohydrate block} = 9 \text{ grams}$$
$$1 \text{ fat block} = 3 \text{ grams}$$

A typical woman needs to eat three blocks each of protein, carbohydrate, and fat at each meal, which means her meal should consist of 21 grams of protein, 27 grams of carbohydrates and 9 grams of fat.

A typical man needs to eat four blocks each of protein, carbohydrate, and fat at every meal, which means his meal should consist of 28 grams of protein, 36 grams of carbohydrate and 12 grams of fat.

A child typically needs two blocks each of protein, carbohydrate, and fat at every meal. That means he or she should eat 14 grams of protein, 18 grams of carbohydrate, and 6 grams of fat at every meal.

On the back of every can or package is a Nutrition Facts Label. Included on the label is information on how many grams of protein, carbohydrate, and fat is found in each serving. When calculating carbohydrates, subtract the dietary fiber content from the total number of carbo-hydrate grams. Don't agonize over making a meal perfect. You'll know an hour or two after the meal if you're in or out of the Zone. Just make the necessary adjustments the next time you eat that exact same meal.

First, take a look at the following chart, which lists many of the con-venience protein products that are on the market. These are handy to add to a frozen dinner or can of soup. All products are not created equal, espe-cially when soy is involved. That makes it important to read the label. For example, the Morningstar Farms Grillers burger has 18 grams of protein and 3 grams of carbohydrate. The Morningstar Farms Garden Veggie patty has only 10 grams of protein and 5 grams of carbohydrate. It's also a good idea to occasionally check the label of old favorites, because compa-nies sometimes change the contents. For example, when the book *The Soy Zone* came out, Morningstar Farms Recipes soy protein crumbles con-tained 12 grams of protein and 2 grams of carbohydrate per ½-cup serving. Today, the same product contains 10 grams of protein and 2 grams of car-bohydrate per ⅔-cup serving.

People on low-sodium diets also have to read the nutritional label carefully.

Let's start with the protein and highlight a few of the many conven-ience protein products.

Boca Sausage	1 sausage = 12 grams protein (8 grams fat)
Home Market Foods Turkey Meatballs	3 meatballs = 14 grams protein (5 grams fat)
Gimme Lean Sausage Style	2 ounces = 8 grams protein (0 grams fat)
Morningstar Farms Breakfast Patty	1 patty = 10 grams protein (3 grams fat)
Morningstar Farms Grillers Veggie Burgers	1 patty = 15 grams protein (6 grams fat)

Morningstar Farms Recipes Crumbles	⅔ cup = 10 grams protein (2.5 grams fat)
Purdue Shortcuts Chicken Breast Roasted Original	½ cup = 17 grams protein (1½ grams fat)
Sonoma Brand Chicken Sausage	1 link = 16 grams protein (7 grams fat)
Veggie Patch Meatless Breakfast Patties	2 patties = 13 grams protein (8 grams fat)
Banquet Grill Chicken Breast Patties (glazed)	1 patty = 15 grams protein (4.5 grams fat)
Yves Veggie Deli Slices	3½ slices = 13 grams protein (0 grams fat)
Trader Joe's Snack Master Turkey Jerky (2.5-ounce package)	1 ounce = 14 grams protein (3 grams carbs)
Tyson Grilled Chicken Strips	1 ounce = 7 grams protein (0 grams fat)

There are a large number of canned and frozen carbohydrate choices. Here are a few examples to get you started. Gram content will vary slightly from brand to brand.

Del Monte Diced Tomatoes (Basil, Garlic, and Oregano)	½ cup = 10 grams carbohydrates
DeMoulas Pepper and Onion Stir-fry (frozen)	16-ounce bag = 10 grams carbohydrates
Del Monte Fresh Cut Zucchini (canned)	½ cup = 6 grams carbohydrates
Del Monte Fresh Cut Italian Beans	14½-ounce can = 10½ grams carbohydrates

Green Giant Cut Green Beans	14½-ounce can = 10½ grams carbohydrates
Mixed Frozen Vegetables	16-ounce bag
Trader Joe Artichoke Salsa	5 tablespoons = 10 grams carbohydrate and 5 grams fat
Campbell's Cream of Chicken Soup (98 percent fat free)	10¾-ounce can = 20 grams carbohydrate (2 grams fat, 7 grams protein)
Campbell's Cream of Mushroom with Roasted Garlic	10¾ ounce can = 25 grams carbohydrate (7 grams fat)
Canned black beans, chickpeas, kidney beans	¼ cup = 9 grams carbohydrate
Applesauce, unsweetened, or Mandarin oranges	⅓ cup = 9 grams carbohydrate
Fruit cocktail or peaches or pineapple, canned in water	½ cup = 9 grams carbohydrate

Now, let's open a can of soup.

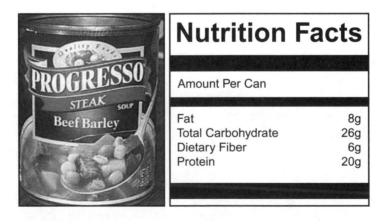

Let's return to the soup we talked about in chapter 1, Progresso Beef Barley. For women, the 20 grams of protein and 8 grams of fat are about right, but 20 grams of carbohydrate aren't enough. Women should add 1 block of carbohydrate, such as ½ cup of grapes or 1 peach. Or open another can, perhaps adding ½ cup diced tomatoes or a generous ½ cup of cut zucchini.

Men should add a block of protein, such as 1 piece of string cheese, 1 ounce of skinless chicken breast, or, from the list of convenience proteins, ⅔ cup soy crumbles, which can be added to the soup before it's heated. Two complete blocks are needed to bring the meal up to 36 grams of carbohydrate. Add an apple or an orange, or ½ cup canned beans. If fruit or beans are selected, a block of fat is also needed for the typical man's lunch. Three olives or 6 peanuts would fit the bill. If the turkey meatballs are added, don't add fat.

A child would eat about three-quarters of the can of soup.

Once you master gramming, you can open virtually any can of soup and know what you have to add to make a complete meal. Make sure to choose soups that contain barley, lentils, or other Zone-favorable vegetables rather than those with noodles or rice.

Now you're ready to graduate to frozen dinners. Have you ever noticed that you get hungry a couple of hours after you have a frozen dinner? That's because you have to add to most of them to eat enough for a full Zone meal.

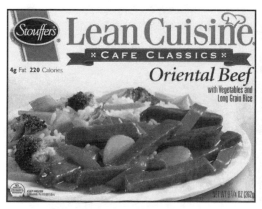

Nutrition Facts

Amount Per Package

Fat	4g
Total Carbohydrate	32g
Dietary `Fiber	2g
Protein	15g

The Stouffer's Lean Cuisine Oriental Beef dinner has 15 grams of protein (2 blocks), 20 grams of carbohydrate (2 blocks), and 4 grams of fat (a little more than 1 block). Women should add 1 protein block, such as 1 ounce of grated cheese on top or 1 block of the convenience proteins listed in the chart above, in addition to 1 block of carbohydrate and 2 blocks of fat. Add a can of Cream of Mushroom Soup cooked in water, which has 9 grams (1 block) carbohydrate and 2.5 grams (1 block) of fat, and six olives (1 block of fat). Or a small side salad (a freebie) topped with ¼ cup chickpeas (1 carbohydrate block) and ⅔ teaspoon olive oil (2 fat blocks) and vinegar dressing to complete the meal.

Men should add 2 blocks of protein, 2 blocks of carbohydrate, and 3 blocks of fat. A piece of low-carbohydrate bread (1 carbohydrate block) spread with 2 tablespoons guacamole (2 fat blocks) topped with 3 ounces deli meat (2 protein blocks), and ½ cup grapes (1 carbohydrate block) add up to a Zone meal.

Or add 2 ounces Tyson Grilled Chicken Strips (2 protein blocks), 1½ cups Del Monte fresh cut zucchini (2 carbohydrate blocks), and a side salad with 1 teaspoon olive oil (3 fat blocks) and vinegar dressing.

Now you see why most TV dinners don't hold you until the next meal.

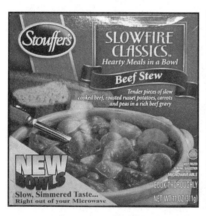

Stouffer's Beef Stew contains 21 grams of protein, 21 grams of carbohydrate, and 12 grams of fat. Women can fly out the door with the dinner and 1 block of carbohydrate, such as ½ apple or ½ cup of grapes. Or they can add a can of green beans or a 16-ounce bag of frozen vegetables (each 1 block). The fat is a tad high, but won't hurt too much. Just have one less block of fat at your next meal. A typical man will need to add 2 blocks of carbohydrate and 1 block of protein. A string cheese (1 protein block) and an apple (2 carbohydrate blocks) will bring the meal into the Zone, or add ½ ounce of turkey jerky (1 protein block) and 1 cup canned peaches packed in water (2 carbohydrate blocks).

A typical child should eat roughly half of the beef stew package.

CAN-DO DINNER EXAMPLES

A quick dinner for two (one man, one woman) can be made simply by opening four cans and adding some protein and fat.

ITEM	PROTEIN	CARBOHYDRATE	FAT
1 14½ can Cut Green Beans		10g	
½ 14½-ounce can Italian Green Beans		5g	
1 10¾-ounce can Cream of Mushroom Soup		22g	5g
1 cup 1-percent milk	8g	11.7g	2.5g
½ cup kidney beans		18g	21

The above ingredients will give the carbohydrate portion for a dinner for two (64 grams, or about 7 blocks). Over medium heat in a nonstick pan, brown your protein choice, such as 7 ounces of cut-up chicken (7 blocks protein, 4 grams fat), in 2 tablespoons olive oil (3 blocks fat). Add the rest of the ingredients. Lower the heat to medium-low and cook, covered, until the chicken is done, stirring occasionally.

Here's another example of a quick can-do dinner:

ITEM	CARBOHYDRATE	FAT
1 10¾-ounce can tomato soup	47g	2g
1 10¾-ounce can French Onion Soup	12g	4½g
1 1-pound bag of Broccoli, Green Beans, Pearl Onions and Peppers	15g	

Remember, a woman needs 27 grams of carbohydrate at each meal and a man needs 36 grams. That just happens to be just about equal to the amount in those two cans and the frozen vegetable. Add your protein choice and some fat blocks, such as olives or olive oil, and it's dinner for two, a quick and easy stew.

The Web is a great place to look for recipes. A lot of simple recipes that can be easily Zoned can be found on Campbell's website, www.campbell-kitchen.com. The website www.reynoldskitchen.com gives a number of quick ways to cook with foil. Not only are the recipes easy, but cleanup time is lessened. One recipe we've tried takes the frozen taste completely out of frozen vegetables. Thai-Style vegetables start with a sheet of Reynolds Wrap Heavy Duty Aluminum Foil. All you do is spray the sheet with nonstick spray, put a 16-ounce package of frozen vegetables on the foil, and sprinkle soy sauce, minced ginger, and lime on the vegetables. Fold the foil to make a packet, allowing room for heat circulation inside.

Cook the vegetables in a 450°F. oven for 20 minutes, or grill 10 to 12 minutes on a covered grill.

Websites also have a number of recipes that feature barley, such as www.albertabarley.com. Under the salads category, the Barley Tabouli, Bean and Barley Salad, and Greek Barley Salad are all very tasty and very Zoneful. Also, don't forget the official Zone diet website, www.drsears.com Hundreds of Zoned recipes for breakfasts, lunches, and dinners can be found in the archives.

LUNCHES

Tuna Marseille

Diane Manteca

Prep: 15 minutes

Yield: 2 (4-block) meals

Block Size	Ingredients
	4 cups shredded romaine lettuce
6 protein, 1 fat	One 6-ounce can tuna in water
1 carbohydrate	1½ cups thawed frozen string beans
¾ carbohydrate	¾ cup sliced roasted peppers
1 carbohydrate	2 ripe tomatoes, sliced
2 carbohydrate	½ cup chickpeas
2 protein, 4 fat	2 ounces soft goat cheese
3 fat	2 teaspoons extra-virgin olive oil
	4 tablespoons tarragon wine vinegar
	Salt and pepper to taste
2½ carbohydrate	2 ounces whole wheat pita, sliced into thin triangles

Instructions

On a large plate, spread the romaine lettuce. In the center, mound the tuna. Place the string beans, peppers, tomatoes, chickpeas, and goat cheese around the tuna. Whisk the olive oil and vinegar in a small bowl and season with salt and pepper. Drizzle over the salad. Serve with the pita triangles.

Asian Sesame Chicken and Cashew Salad

Diane Manteca

Prep: 15 minutes   **Yield:** 2 (4-block) servings

Block Size	Ingredients
	3 tablespoons soy sauce
2 fat	1⅓ teaspoons toasted sesame oil
8 protein, 2 fat	8 ounces Perdue cooked skinless chicken breast, cut into 1-inch pieces
	1½ cups fresh bean sprouts
1 carbohydrate	2 whole red peppers, julienned
2 carbohydrate	⅔ cup canned, sliced water chestnuts
1 carbohydrate	2 cups frozen string beans, defrosted
4 carbohydrate	1 cup cooked, chilled barley
	Salt and pepper to taste
	4 cups shredded romaine lettuce
2 fat	8 toasted cashews, chopped
	3 scallions (green onions), chopped fine

Instructions

In a large bowl, add the soy sauce and sesame oil and blend well. Toss in the chicken, bean sprouts, peppers, water chestnuts, string beans, and barley. Season with a little salt and pepper. Divide the lettuce between 2 plates and top with the salad. Garnish with the cashews and scallions.

Baked Chili Chicken Rellenos with Corn Tortilla

Diane Manteca

Prep: 15 minutes
Cooking: 40 minutes

Yield: 2 (4-block) servings

Blocks	Ingredients
1 carbohydrate	10 ounces chopped frozen peppers
1 carbohydrate	1½ cups chopped frozen onion
	Kosher salt and pepper to taste
4 protein, 1 fat	⅔ cup Perdue Shortcuts Chicken Breast, Roasted Original
3 fat	2 tablespoons light sour cream
4 carbohydrate	1 cup canned black beans
	1 teaspoon Cajun spices (Emeril or Paul Prudhomme)
2 protein	½ cup liquid egg white product
2 protein, 2 fat	3½ slices Kraft low-fat sharp cheddar, cut into strips
2 carbohydrate	2 corn tortillas, cut into 2-inch strips
2 fat	12 olives

Instructions

1 Preheat the oven to 350°F. Spray an 8- or 9-inch baking dish with olive oil cooking spray.

2 Spray a nonstick skillet with olive oil cooking spray and heat it over medium heat. Sauté the peppers and onions with a sprinkle of kosher salt and pepper until the onions are softened, about 5 minutes. Add the chicken, sour cream, black beans, olives, and Cajun spices and cook for 1 minute. Place this mixture evenly in the baking dish. Pour the egg product on top and bake for 25 minutes, or until the eggs are firm. Place the strips of cheese and tortilla strips on top and bake 8 to 10 minutes, or until the cheese is melted and the tortilla strips are golden.

Crab-Stuffed Portobello Mushrooms with Cherry Tomato Salad

Diane Manteca

Prep: 10 minutes
Cooking: 15 minutes

Yield: 2 (4-block) servings

Block Size	Ingredients
Mushrooms	
2 carbohydrate	1½ pounds fresh portobello mushroom, stems removed
3 protein, 3 fat	¾ cup shredded part-skim mozzarella
1 carbohydrate	½ cup drained and chopped roasted peppers
2 carbohydrate	½ cup dark red kidney beans, drained, rinsed and chopped
5 protein, 2 fat	7 ounces canned crabmeat
	1 tablespoon dried oregano
	½ cup chopped frozen onion
	1 tablespoon chopped jarred garlic, rinsed
Cherry Tomato Salad	
1 carbohydrate	2 cups cherry tomatoes
2 carbohydrate	½ cup canned chickpeas, rinsed
3 fat	8 tablespoons Wish-Bone Creamy Lite Italian Dressing
	Shredded romaine lettuce

Instructions

1 Preheat the oven to 425°F. Spray olive oil cooking spray in a baking dish. Wipe the mushrooms clean and place them upside down in the baking dish. In a medium bowl, combine the remaining ingredients and stuff the mushrooms with the mixture. Bake 15 to 20 minutes or until golden brown and bubbly.

2 In a medium bowl, combine the cherry tomatoes, chickpeas, and dressing. Serve on the lettuce with the mushrooms on the side.

Roast Turkey Salad and Citrus-Chive Vinaigrette

Diane Manteca

Prep: 15 minutes

Yield: 2 (4-block) servings

Block Size	Ingredients
8 protein, 2 fat	8 ounces unsliced deli roast turkey breast, cut into 1-inch cubes
1½ carbohydrate	2½ cups frozen Green Giant sugar snap peas, thawed
2 carbohydrate	1 cup grapes
3 carbohydrate	¾ cup canned chickpeas, drained
½ carbohydrate	1 red bell pepper, cut into 1-inch pieces
1 carbohydrate	⅓ cup orange juice
6 fat	4 teaspoons extra-virgin olive oil
	1 tablespoon balsamic vinegar
	½ teaspoon kosher salt
	½ teaspoon black pepper
	1 bunch fresh chives, chopped fine
	3 cups baby spinach

Instructions

In a large bowl, combine the turkey, snap peas, grapes, chickpeas, and red pepper. In a small bowl, combine the orange juice, olive oil, balsamic vinegar, salt, and pepper. Whisk until well blended. Add the chives and mix well. Divide the spinach onto 2 dinner plates. Place the turkey salad on each and drizzle with the citrus-chive dressing.

Indian Curried Chicken and Yogurt Salad with Lentils

Diane Manteca

Prep: 15 minutes   **Yield:**   2 (4-block) servings

Block Size	Ingredients
2 protein, 2 carbohydrate	1 cup Dannon nonfat plain yogurt
	2 tablespoons curry powder
	½ teaspoon kosher or sea salt
6 protein, 2 fat	1⅓ cups Perdue Shortcuts cooked chicken strips
4 carbohydrate	2 cups cooked lentils
1 carbohydrate	2 cups cherry tomatoes, cut in half
1 carbohydrate	½ cup Del Monte lite apricots, drained and cut in half
	2 or 3 scallions (green onions), chopped
	Lettuce leaves
6 fat	24 crushed cashews

Instructions

In a large mixing bowl, combine the yogurt, curry powder, and salt and mix well. Add the chicken, lentils, cherry tomatoes, apricots, and scallions and toss. Serve the salad on the lettuce leaves and garnish with crushed cashews.

Lentil and Chicken Sausage Soup

Diana Manteca

Prep: 10 minutes
Cooking: 10 minutes

Yield: 2 (4-block) servings

Block Size	Ingredients
5 fat, 6 protein	5 sun-dried tomato and basil chicken sausages
3 carbohydrate, 1 fat, 2 protein	3 cups Progresso Lentil Soup
1 carbohydrate	1 cup diced tomatoes
1 carbohydrate	½ cup drained and chopped roasted peppers
	1 tablespoon chopped jarred garlic, rinsed
2 fat	12 olives, chopped
3 carbohydrate	1 cup canned light fruit cocktail

Instructions

1 Spray a nonstick sauté pan with olive oil cooking spray and cook the sausages over medium-low heat, turning occasionally, until done in the center, about 10 minutes. Cut the sausages into ½-inch slices. In a saucepan, combine the lentil soup, tomatoes, roasted peppers, garlic, olives, and cooked sausages. Bring to a boil, lower the heat, and cook for 5 minutes, or until heated through.

2 Serve the fruit cocktail for dessert.

Smoked Salmon and Baby Green Sandwich with Herbal Tomato Soup

Diane Manteca

Prep: 10 minutes   **Yield:**   2 (4-block) servings
Cooking: 5 minutes

Block Size	**Ingredients**
Herbal Tomato Soup	
2 carbohydrate	1 cup Del Monte diced tomatoes with basil, garlic, and oregano, with juices
	1 cup fat-free chicken stock
	½ teaspoon dried basil
	½ teaspoon dried oregano
	Salt and pepper
Smoked Salmon Sandwiches	
	2 cups baby greens
3 fat	2 teaspoons extra-virgin olive oil
	Kosher salt and black pepper
8 protein, 3 fat	12 ounces smoked salmon
2 fat	½ medium avocado, pitted, peeled, and sliced thin
2 carbohydrate	1 cup roasted peppers, drained, patted dry, and sliced
	2 tablespoons thinly sliced red onions
4 carbohydrate	4 slices Pepperidge Farm multigrain 7 light bread

Instructions

1 To make the soup, in a medium saucepan, bring all the soup ingredients to a boil. Season with salt and pepper.

2 To make the sandwiches, in a medium bowl, toss the baby greens with the olive oil, and season with salt and pepper. Layer the salmon, avocado, roasted peppers, baby greens, and onions on the bread to make sandwiches.

Roast Turkey Reuben with Tossed Green Salad and Olives

Diane Manteca

Prep: 10 minutes

Yield: 2 (4-block) servings

Block Size	Ingredients
Sandwiches	
4 carbohydrate	4 slices Pepperidge Farm multigrain 7 light bread, toasted
	Dijon mustard
5 protein	5 ounces fat-free roast turkey breast
3 protein	3 ounces Alpine Lace Fat-free Swiss Cheese
	½ cup canned sauerkraut
4 fat	5 tablespoons Wish-Bone Lite Thousand Island Dressing
Tossed Salad	
	4 cups romaine lettuce
2 fat	4 teaspoons slivered toasted almonds
	Hellman's Fat-Free Caesar Dressing
2 fat	12 queen-size stuffed olives
Fruit	
2 carbohydrate	2 fresh peaches, sliced
2 carbohydrate	1 cup fresh or thawed frozen blueberries
	Dash of cinnamon

Instructions

1 Place a slice of bread on each of two plates. Spread the bread with Dijon mustard and layer on the turkey, Swiss cheese, sauerkraut, and Thousand Island dressing. Top each with another slice of bread.

2 In a medium bowl, toss together the salad ingredients.

3 In a small bowl, mix the peaches, blueberries, and cinnamon.

4 Serve the sandwiches and salads together, with the fruit for dessert.

DINNERS

Pesto Sole with Barley Primavera

Diane Manteca

Prep: 12 minutes
Cooking: 15 minutes

Yield: 2 (4-block) servings

Block Size	Ingredients
	1 tablespoon chopped jarred garlic, rinsed
	2 tablespoons dried **or** 6 tablespoons finely chopped fresh basil
5½ fat	3⅔ teaspoons extra-virgin olive oil
	Kosher salt and pepper to taste
1 carbohydrate	1½ cups chopped frozen onions
2 carbohydrate	4 cups Green Giant San Francisco frozen vegetables
4 carbohydrate	1 cup cooked barley
1 carbohydrate	4 ounces dry white wine
	1 cup fat-free chicken or fish stock
8 protein, 4½ fat	12 ounces sole or flounder

Instructions

1 Spray a 9 x 12-inch baking dish with olive oil cooking spray. Preheat the oven to 350°F.

2 To make the pesto, in a small bowl combine 1½ teaspoons of the garlic, basil, and olive oil. Add a dash of salt and pepper.

3 Spray a nonstick sauté pan with olive oil cooking spray and heat over high heat. Add the onions, vegetables, and remaining 1½ teaspoons garlic and sauté for 5 minutes, or until tender yet firm. Stir in the barley, wine, and stock. Spread the vegetable mixture in the baking dish and layer the fish on top. Spread the fish with the pesto. Bake for 12 to 15 minutes, or until the fish is firm to the touch.

Caribbean Roast Salmon with Salsa Topping on a Bed of Black Beans and Vegetables

Diane Manteca

Prep: 12 minutes   **Yield:**   2 (4-block) servings
Cooking: 15 minutes

Block Size	Ingredients
Vegetables	
5 fat	3⅓ teaspoons olive oil
	2 teaspoons chopped jarred garlic, drained and rinsed
2 carbohydrate	4 cups Green Giant San Francisco frozen vegetables
	2 tablespoons Cajun spice mix (Emeril or Paul Prudomme)
5 carbohydrate	1¼ cups black beans, drained
	Juice of 2 limes
	Kosher salt and pepper to taste
Salmon	
8 protein, 3 fat	Two 6-ounce salmon fillets
1 carbohydrate	½ cup Old El Paso Homestyle Salsa
	2 scallions (green onions), chopped

Instructions

1 Preheat the oven to 400°F and spray olive oil cooking spray on a cookie sheet.

2 In a nonstick skillet, heat the olive oil and sauté the garlic, vegetables, and 1 tablespoon of the Cajun spices until the vegetables are tender. Stir in the black beans and heat through. Stir in the lime juice and season with kosher salt and pepper. Keep the mixture warm.

3 Place the salmon fillets on the cookie sheet and sprinkle the remaining 1 tablespoon Cajun spices on top. Bake 15 minutes, or until the salmon is done as desired. Divide the vegetables between 2 dinner plates and lay the salmon fillets on top. Garnish with the salsa and scallions.

New England Baked Salmon "Pie" with Clam Sauce and BBQ Beans

Diane Manteca

Prep: 8 minutes
Cooking: 20 minutes

Yield: 2 (4-block) servings

Block Size	Ingredients
7 protein, 2½ fat	10½ ounces salmon fillet, divided in half
1 carbohydrate	4 fat-free saltine crackers
2½ fat	1⅔ teaspoons olive oil
1 protein, 2 carbohydrate, 3 fat	¾ cup Pepperidge Farm Clam Chowder
4 carbohydrate	1 cup dark kidney beans, drained
1 carbohydrate	2 tablespoon hickory-smoked BBQ sauce

Instructions

1 Preheat the oven to 400°F and spray a 9 x 12-inch baking dish with nonstick cooking spray. Place the salmon in the baking dish and bake for 10 minutes.

2 Meanwhile, in a small bowl, crush the crackers and sprinkle with the olive oil. In a small saucepan over medium-low heat, warm the chowder. Pour the chowder over the salmon and sprinkle with the crushed saltines. Bake for 10 minutes more, or until cracker crumbs are lightly golden.

3 In a separate small saucepan, warm the beans and the BBQ sauce. Serve with the salmon.

Thai Coconut Curried Haddock Baked in Foil

Diane Manteca

Prep: 10 minutes
Cooking: 15 to 20 minutes

Yield: 2 (4-block) servings

Block Size	Ingredients
Haddock	
8 protein, 3 fat	12 ounces haddock fillets
1 carbohydrate	Juice of 2 limes
	2 tablespoons curry powder
	1 tablespoon chopped fresh ginger
4 carbohydrate	2 cups diced canned pineapple in water, drained
	2 scallions (green onions), chopped
Vegetables	
5 fat	3⅓ teaspoons olive oil
1 carbohydrate	½ of a 16-ounce bag dry coleslaw mix
	1 tablespoon chopped jarred garlic, rinsed
2 carbohydrate	1 bag frozen Green Giant Japanese Teriyaki vegetable mix
	Salt and black pepper

Instructions

1 Preheat the oven to 400°F.

2 Place a 24 × 24-inch piece of aluminum foil on a baking sheet. Lay the haddock on the sheet and sprinkle it with the lime juice, curry powder, and ginger. Top with the pineapple and spray lightly with olive oil cooking spray. Bring the sides of the foil up and crimp the top of the foil together above the haddock. Bake for 15 to 20 minutes.

3 Meanwhile, in a nonstick skillet over medium heat, heat the olive oil. Add the coleslaw mix and garlic and sauté for 5 minutes, or until the cabbage is softened. Add the vegetables and cook for another 4 to 5 minutes, or until tender yet firm. Season with salt and pepper.

4 Divide the vegetables between 2 serving plates. Carefully open the top of the foil, remove the haddock with a spatula, and place the haddock on top of the vegetables. Garnish with the scallions.

Peking Shrimp

Diane Manteca

Prep: 10 minutes
Cooking: 15 minutes

Yield: 2 (4-block) servings

Block Size	Ingredients

Shrimp and Vegetables

Block Size	Ingredients
4 fat	2⅔ teaspoons light olive oil
	1 tablespoon chopped jarred garlic, rinsed
1 carbohydrate	One 16-ounce bag Oriental frozen vegetable mix, thawed
1 carbohydrate	⅓ cup canned sliced water chestnuts, drained
8 protein, 1½ fat	12 ounces raw large shrimp, peeled and deveined
	Salt and pepper to taste
4 carbohydrate	1 cup cooked barley
2½ fat	24 crushed dry roasted peanuts

Sauce

Block Size	Ingredients
1 carbohydrate	4 teaspoons cornstarch
1 carbohydrate	2 teaspoons fructose powder
	4 tablespoon soy sauce
	½ cup chicken stock

Instructions

1 In a nonstick skillet over high heat, heat half the oil. Add the garlic, mixed vegetables, and water chestnuts and stir-fry 2 to 3 minutes. Remove the vegetables and set aside in a bowl.

2 Heat the remaining oil over high heat. Add the shrimp and stir-fry 3 to 4 minutes, or until the shrimp turn pink. Return the cooked vegetables to the pan. Add salt and pepper to taste.

3 In a small bowl, combine the sauce ingredients. Blend well. Stir the sauce into the shrimp-vegetable mixture and heat on high until bubbly.

4 Divide the barley between 2 plates. Serve the shrimp-vegetable mixture on top of the barley and top with the peanuts.

Scallops St. Jacques with Roasted Asparagus

Diane Manteca

Prep: 15 minutes   **Yield:**   2 (4-block) servings
Cooking: 15 minutes

Block Size	Ingredients
Scallops	
1 protein, 1 carbohydrate, 1 fat	1 cup low-fat milk
1 carbohydrate	4 teaspoons cornstarch
7 protein, 2 fat	10 ounces bay scallops (the small ones)
1 carbohydrate	½ cup dry white wine
	2 tablespoons chopped jarred garlic, rinsed
1 carbohydrate	2½ cups Green Giant canned sliced mushrooms, drained
1 carbohydrate	1 tablespoon Progresso lemon-herb bread crumbs
Asparagus	
1 carbohydrate	24 fresh asparagus spears
1 carbohydrate	10 ounces chopped frozen peppers
5 fat	3⅓ teaspoons extra-virgin olive oil
	Salt and pepper to taste
	Lemon juice
1 carbohydrate	½ cup grapes

Instructions

1 Preheat the oven to 400°F. In a small bowl, combine the milk and cornstarch. Spray a 9 x 9-inch baking dish with olive oil cooking spray. Place the scallops in the dish in one layer. In a small saucepan, bring the wine and garlic to a low boil over medium-low heat for 3 minutes. Turn the heat to low and whisk in the milk/cornstarch mixture. Whisk and cook until thickened, about 5 minutes, and add the mushrooms. Pour the mixture over the scallops, sprinkle with the bread crumbs, and bake for 15 minutes, or until golden and bubbly.

2 Meanwhile, to make the asparagus, wash the stalks and snap off the tough bottom portion. Dry the stalks and toss them with the peppers, olive oil, salt, and pepper. Place the vegetables in a single layer on a baking sheet and roast them with the scallops for about 12 minutes, or until tender. Drizzle on the lemon juice.

3 Serve the asparagus with the scallops, and serve the grapes for dessert.

Baked Shrimp Palermo with Sicilian Chickpea Salad

Diane Manteca

Prep: 10 minutes
Cooking: 12 minutes

Yield: 2 (4-block) servings

Block Size	Ingredients
Shrimp	
8 protein, 2 fat	12 ounces raw medium shrimp, shelled and deveined
	1 tablespoon chopped jarred garlic, rinsed
	1 tablespoon dried basil
	1 tablespoon dried oregano
	Kosher or sea salt to taste
	¼ teaspoon red pepper chili flakes
2 carbohydrate	1 cup Del Monte canned tomatoes diced with basil, garlic, and oregano, with juices
1 fat	6 manzilla stuffed olives, cut in half
Chickpea Salad	
4 carbohydrate	1 cup canned chickpeas, drained
	½ cup thawed frozen mixed peppers
	1 teaspoon dried basil
	Salt and pepper to taste
2 carbohydrate	1 cup grapes
4 fat	3 tablespoons Wish-Bone Caesar Olive Oil Lite dressing
1 fat	1 tablespoon toasted pine nuts
	2 romaine lettuce leaves

Instructions

1 Spray a nonstick skillet with olive oil cooking spray and add the shrimp, garlic, basil, oregano, salt, and chili flakes. Cook over high heat for 2 to 3 minutes, or until the shrimp have turned pink. Add the tomatoes and olives and bring to a quick boil for 2 to 3 minutes, or until the sauce has reached the desired consistency.

2 Mix the salad ingredients (except the lettuce) in a large bowl. Place the salad on the lettuce leaves and serve with the shrimp.

Chinese Egg Foo Yong

Diane Manteca

Prep: 10 minutes
Cooking: 15 minutes

Yield: 2 (4-block) servings

Block Size	Ingredients
5 fat	3⅓ teaspoon olive oil
	1 tablespoon chopped jarred garlic, rinsed
	2 tablespoons frozen chopped onion
1 carbohydrate	One 16-ounce bag thawed frozen Oriental vegetables
	2 cups canned bean sprouts
	4 tablespoons soy sauce
	Salt and pepper to taste
3 carbohydrate	¾ cup canned white navy beans, drained and rinsed
8 protein	2 cups liquid egg white product
4 carbohydrate, 6 fat	2 cups condensed Cream of Mushroom soup
	Toasted sesame seeds for garnish
	Chives or scallions (green onions) for garnish

Instructions

1 In a nonstick skillet over medium-high heat, heat the oil and sauté the garlic and onions until the onions are translucent, about 3 minutes. Add the Oriental vegetables, bean sprouts, 1 tablespoon of the soy sauce, and a pinch of salt and pepper and cook on high heat for 2 minutes, or until the vegetables are softened. Add the navy beans, lower the heat to medium, and pour the egg product on top of the vegetables. Let the eggs cook, not stirring, until they have set like an omelet, about 10 minutes. Placing a cover over the pan helps the top to set.

2 Meanwhile, in a small saucepan over medium heat, combine the mushroom soup and the remaining 3 tablespoons soy sauce and heat until warmed.

3 Cut the egg foo yong in half and, using a spatula, place each half on a dinner plate. Top with the sauce, garnish with the sesame seeds and chives or scallion (green onions), and serve.

Teriyaki Steak with Sautéed Oriental Vegetables

Diane Manteca

Prep: 10 minutes   **Yield:**   2 (4-block) servings
Cooking: 20 minutes

Block Size	Ingredients
1 carbohydrate	2 teaspoons fructose powder
	4 tablespoons Kikkoman teriyaki sauce
8 protein, 5 fat	8 ounces beef round steak
3 fat	2 teaspoons light olive oil
	1 tablespoon chopped jarred garlic
	1 tablespoon chopped fresh ginger
1 carbohydrate	One 16-ounce bag frozen Oriental vegetables
2 carbohydrate	⅔ cup water chestnuts
1 carbohydrate	2½ cups Green Giant sliced, canned mushrooms
	Kosher salt and pepper to taste
2 carbohydrate	1 cup cut pineapple
1 carbohydrate	1 cup sliced fresh strawberries

Instructions

1 In a small saucepan, combine the fructose powder and teriyaki sauce. Cook over medium heat for 1 minute, whisking constantly.

2 Place the steak under a broiler or on an outdoor grill and cook for 10 minutes, or until no longer pink in the center.

3 In a nonstick sauté pan over high heat, heat the olive oil. Add the garlic and ginger and sauté for 15 seconds. Add the frozen vegetables, water chestnuts, and mushrooms and cook 10 minutes, or until tender and heated through. Season with salt and pepper.

4 Place the steaks on 2 plates and top with the teriyaki sauce. Serve with the vegetables. Serve the fruit for dessert.

Spanish Seafood Stew

Diane Manteca

Prep: 10 minutes   **Yield:**   2 (4-block) servings
Cooking: 15 minutes

Block Size	Ingredients
6½ fat	4⅓ teaspoons extra-virgin olive oil
	2 tablespoons chopped jarred garlic, rinsed
1 carbohydrate	½ cup drained, chopped roasted peppers
	1 teaspoon dried thyme
	1 teaspoon sweet paprika
	½ teaspoon saffron
	Kosher salt and black pepper to taste
	One 8-ounce bottle clam juice or 1 cup fat-free chicken stock
1 carbohydrate	½ cup dry white wine
	1 bay leaf
2 carbohydrate	1 cup canned Del Monte Italian-style diced tomatoes, with juice
1 carbohydrate	1½ cups cut frozen string beans
1 carbohydrate	One 9-ounce package frozen Bird's Eye artichoke hearts, thawed
2 carbohydrate	½ cup canned chickpeas, drained and rinsed
6 protein, 1 fat	9 ounces fresh haddock
2 protein, ½ fat	3 ounces uncooked shrimp, peeled and deveined

Instructions

In a large sauté pan, heat the olive oil and sauté the garlic and roasted peppers over medium heat until just heated through, about 2 minutes. Add the thyme, paprika, saffron, ½ teaspoon kosher salt, and a pinch of black pepper and cook on high for 2 minutes, stirring constantly. Add the clam juice or stock, white wine, and bay leaf and bring to a boil for 1 minute. Add the tomatoes, string beans, artichoke hearts, and chickpeas and cook for 1 minute. Lower the heat to medium and add the haddock and shrimp, pushing the fish carefully to submerse it in the liquid. Cover and cook 2 minutes. Uncover, carefully flip the haddock and shrimp over, and cook, uncovered, for 10 minutes, or until the haddock is flaky and fully cooked. Season with salt and pepper and serve.

Pork Sauerbraten with Sauerkraut and Roasted Brussels Sprouts

Diana Manteca

Prep: 15 minutes
Cooking: 25 minutes

Yield: 2 (4-block) servings

Block Size	Ingredients
Pork Sauerbraten	
½ carbohydrate	¾ cup chopped frozen onion
1 carbohydrate	1 cup canned Green Giant LaSuer baby carrots, drained
½ carbohydrate	One 10-ounce bag frozen cauliflower
1 carbohydrate	1 cup canned sauerkraut, drained
2 carbohydrate	3 low-fat gingersnaps, crushed into crumbs
	2 cups fat-free beef broth
1 carbohydrate	4 teaspoons cornstarch
	1 teaspoon caraway seeds
	2 tablespoons tomato paste
	1 teaspoon ground ginger
1 carbohydrate	2 teaspoons fructose
8 protein, 5 fat	8 ounces Hormel cooked pork roast
Brussels Sprouts	
1 carbohydrate	One 16-ounce bag thawed frozen Brussels sprouts
	1 teaspoon kosher salt
	½ teaspoon black pepper
3 fat	2 teaspoons extra-virgin olive oil

Instructions

1 Preheat the oven to 350°F.

2 In a large bowl, combine all the sauerbraten ingredients except the pork. Place the pork in a baking dish and pour mixed ingredients over it. Cover and bake 25 minutes, or until the center is hot. Uncover and bake 5 minutes. Keep the dish warm while you prepare the Brussels sprouts.

3 Increase the oven temperature to 425°F. In a medium bowl, toss the Brussels sprouts, salt, pepper, and olive oil. Place in a 9 × 12-inch baking pan and roast 15 minutes, or until tender. Serve with the sauerbraten.

Shrimp and Cucumber Salad with Spicy Peanut Sauce

Diana Manteca

Prep: 10 minutes   **Yield:**   2 (4-block) servings

Block Size	**Ingredients**
8 protein, 2 fat	12 ounces cooked shrimp
2 carbohydrate	1 cup cooked barley
6 fat, 2 carbohydrate	6 tablespoons House of Tsang Peanut Sauce
	2 cups shredded Chinese (napa) cabbage or lettuce
2 carbohydrate	3 medium cucumbers, peeled, sliced, and cut into ¼-inch rounds
1 carbohydrate	2 red peppers, thinly sliced
	½ bunch scallions (green onions), chopped
1 carbohydrate	⅓ cup canned plums, drained and sliced

Instructions

In a medium bowl, toss the shrimp and barley in the peanut sauce. Divide the cabbage or lettuce on two plates. Place the cucumbers on top, then the shrimp and barley mixture. Garnish the salads with the red peppers, scallion (green onions), and plums.

Zone Basil Pesto

Diane Manteca

This pesto is a great topping on fish or poultry and also can be added to vegetables or used as a dip for vegetables. Try it on spaghetti squash! (One cup of the squash equals one block of carbohydrate.)

Prep: 5 minutes

Yield: 4 (1-block) servings

Block Size	**Ingredients**
2 fat	1 tablespoon toasted pine nuts
2 protein	7 tablespoons grated nonfat Italian Parmesan cheese
2 protein, 2 fat	4 ounces firm tofu
4 carbohydrate	1 cup canned cannellini (white kidney) beans, drained and rinsed
	4 cups fresh basil
	½ cup water
	1 tablespoon chopped jarred garlic
	¼ teaspoon black pepper

Instructions

In a blender or food processor, pulverize the pine nuts. Add the rest of the ingredients and blend until smooth. The pesto can be divided into portions and frozen.

Zone Roasted Red Pepper Pesto

Diane Manteca

This pesto is wonderful on fish, meat, poultry, sandwiches, and vegetables, and is also great as a dip.

Prep: 5 minutes

Yield: 4 (1-block) servings

Block Size	Ingredients
2 fat	8 toasted cashews
4 carbohydrate	2 cups jarred, roasted red peppers, drained
2 protein	7 tablespoons grated imported nonfat Parmesan cheese
2 protein, 2 fat	4 ounces firm tofu
	1 tablespoon dried basil
	1 tablespoon chopped jarred garlic
	¼ teaspoon black pepper

Instructions

In a blender or food processor, pulverize the cashews. Add the remaining ingredients and blend until smooth. This pesto can be divided into portions and frozen.

Chicken Minestrone

Diane Manteca

Prep: 5 minutes   **Yield:**   2 (4-block) servings
Cooking: 10 minutes

Block Size	Ingredients
5 fat	3⅓ teaspoons extra-virgin olive oil
1 carbohydrate	1½ cups frozen cut green beans
	1 teaspoon dried basil
	1 teaspoon dried oregano
	1 tablespoon chopped jarred garlic, rinsed
8 protein, 3 fat	1¾ cups Perdue Shortcuts Chicken Breast, Roasted Original, chopped
3 carbohydrate	1½ cups Classico Basil Marinara Sauce
2 carbohydrate	½ cup red kidney beans, drained and rinsed
2 carbohydrate	One 15-ounce can Del Monte canned stewed Italian-style zucchini
	2 cups fat-free chicken stock
	½ teaspoon kosher salt
	½ teaspoon pepper

Instructions

In a large saucepan over high heat, heat the olive oil. Add the green beans, basil, oregano, and garlic and sauté for 2 minutes. Add the rest of the ingredients and bring to a boil. Lower the heat to medium and simmer for 3 to 4 minutes, or until hot and bubbling.

Chicken and Barley Risotto with Asparagus and Sun-Dried Tomatoes

Diane Manteca

This dish is wonderful served with a romaine salad with a squeeze of lemon juice or balsamic vinegar.

Prep: 10 minutes

Cooking: 10 minutes

Yield: 2 (4-block) servings

Block Size	Ingredients
1 carbohydrate	1½ cups chopped frozen onions
	1 teaspoon chopped jarred garlic, rinsed
	1 tablespoon dried basil
	½ teaspoon kosher or sea salt
1 carbohydrate, 5½ fat	6 sun-dried tomatoes packed in oil, chopped
	4 cups no-fat chicken stock
1 carbohydrate	½ cup white wine
	2 or 3 pinches saffron (optional)
7 protein, 2½ fat	1½ cups Perdue Shortcuts Chicken Breast, Roasted Original, cut up
4 carbohydrate	1 cup cooked barley
1 carbohydrate	2½ cups canned asparagus, drained and cut up
1 protein	3 tablespoons no-fat grated Parmesan cheese
	Salt and pepper (optional)

Instructions

Spray olive oil cooking spray in a nonstick skillet. Add the onions, garlic, basil, and salt and cook over medium-low heat 5 minutes, or until the onion is softened. Add the sun-dried tomatoes, stock, wine, and saffron and bring to a boil for 3 minutes. Raise the heat to medium, add the chicken and barley, and cook 3 to 4 minutes. Add the asparagus and cook for 2 minutes, or until heated through. Add the cheese and season with pepper and salt if needed.

Old-Fashioned Chicken Pot "Pie"

Diane Manteca

Prep: 5 minutes   **Yield:**   2 (4-block) servings
Cooking: 20 minutes

Block Size	Ingredients
7 protein, 2½ fat	1½ cups Perdue Shortcuts Chicken Breast, Roasted Original, cut into 1-inch pieces
1 carbohydrate	1½ cups chopped frozen onions
1 carbohydrate	10 ounces frozen Green Giant mixed vegetables
1 protein, 2 fat, 2 carbohydrate	2 cups Campbell's condensed Cream of Chicken Soup
	½ teaspoon dried sage
	½ teaspoon dried thyme
3½ fat	2⅓ teaspoons olive oil
	Kosher salt and pepper to taste
2 carbohydrate	8 Devonshire Grain Melba Toasts
2 carbohydrate	2 peaches

Instructions

Preheat the oven to 425°F. In a large mixing bowl, combine the chicken, onions, vegetables, soup, spices, oil, and a dash each of kosher salt and pepper. Pour the mixture into a 9 × 12-inch baking dish and bake for 20 minutes, or until hot in the center. Serve topped with the Melba toasts. Serve the peaches on the side.

French Country Cassoulet

Diane Manteca

Prep: 10 minutes
Cooking: 20 minutes

Yield: 2 (4-block) servings

Block Size	Ingredients
5 fat	3⅓ teaspoons extra-virgin olive oil
	2 tablespoons chopped jarred garlic, rinsed
1 carbohydrate	½ cup dry white wine
6 protein, 2 fat	6 ounces Perdue Shortcuts Chicken Breast, Roasted Original, cut into thirds
2 protein, 1 fat	6 slices Oscar Mayer Healthy Favorites sliced ham, cut into 2-inch pieces
4 carbohydrate	1 cup white navy beans, drained
2 carbohydrate	1 cup Del Monte canned diced tomatoes
1 carbohydrate	1 cup canned baby carrots
	2 bay leaves
	1 teaspoon dried whole thyme leaves
	½ teaspoon liquid hickory smoke
	Chopped fresh parsley for garnish

Instructions

In a nonstick skillet over medium heat, heat the olive oil and sauté the garlic 1 minute, just until lightly golden. Add the wine and cook 2 minutes, stirring constantly. Add the remaining ingredients and simmer 15 minutes, or until the sauce is the desired consistency. Garnish with the parsley.

Rosemary and Citrus-Roasted Chicken Breast with Roman Zucchini and Bean Sauté

Diane Manteca

Prep: 10 minutes   **Yield:**   2 (4-block) servings
Cooking: 25 minutes

Block Size	Ingredients
Chicken	
1 carbohydrate	1 lemon, sliced
2 carbohydrate	1 orange, sliced
8 protein, 2 fat	8 ounces boneless skinless chicken breasts
2 fat	1⅛ teaspoons extra-virgin olive oil
	1 tablespoon dried rosemary
	Kosher or sea salt and black pepper
Zucchini and Bean Sauté	
4 fat	2⅔ teaspoons extra-virgin olive oil
	1 tablespoon chopped jarred garlic, rinsed
2 carbohydrate	½ cup dark kidney beans, drained
2 carbohydrate	1 cup Del Monte diced tomatoes with basil, garlic, and oregano, with juices
1 carbohydrate	1 cup Del Monte Italian-style zucchini, not drained

Instructions

1 To make the chicken, preheat the oven to 375°F. Spray an 8 × 8-inch baking dish with olive oil cooking spray. Layer the lemon and orange slices in the dish. Place the chicken breasts on top and drizzle with the olive oil. Sprinkle with the rosemary, salt, and pepper. Bake 25 minutes or until the chicken is fully cooked.

2 Meanwhile, to make the zucchini and bean sauté, in a nonstick skillet over medium-high heat, add the olive oil and sauté the garlic and kidney beans for 2 minutes. Add the tomatoes and zucchini, turn the heat to high, and cook 3 to 4 minutes, or until the zucchini is crisp-tender. Serve with the chicken.

Pollo Puttanesca with Sautéed String Beans

Diane Manteca

Prep: 8 minutes   **Yield:**   2 (4-block) servings
Cooking: 20 minutes

Block Size	Ingredients
Pollo Puttanesca	
3 fat	2 teaspoons olive oil
7 protein, 1½ fat	7 ounces fresh boneless, skinless chicken breasts
1 carbohydrate	1½ cups chopped frozen onions
	1 tablespoon chopped jarred garlic, drained
	2 tablespoons dried oregano
	3 tablespoons capers, drained
4 carbohydrate	2 cups Classico di Napoli jarred tomato sauce
2 fat	12 Progresso oil-cured olives, pitted and halved
	¼ teaspoon red chili pepper flakes (or to taste)
1 protein, 1½ fat	6 anchovies, drained and chopped
String Beans	
2 carbohydrate	3 cups frozen whole string beans, thawed
1 carbohydrate	2½ cups canned or jarred Green Giant pearl onions
	Kosher or sea salt and pepper to taste

Instructions

1 To make the pollo puttanesca, in a nonstick skillet over medium heat, heat the oil. Add the chicken and brown it lightly, 3 to 4 minutes on each side. Add the onions, garlic, oregano, and capers and cook for 1 minute. Pour in the tomato sauce, olives, red pepper, and anchovies. Cook on medium, turning the chicken occasionally, for 10 minutes, or until the chicken is done.

2 To make the string beans, spray a heavy skillet with olive oil cooking spray, add the string beans and onions, and sauté over high heat until the beans are tender and the onions are translucent, 2 to 3 minutes. Season with salt and pepper and serve with the chicken.

Grilled Chicken "Lasagna"

Diane Manteca

Prep: 10 minutes
Cooking: 30 minutes

Yield: 2 (4-block) servings

Block size	Ingredients
1 carbohydrate	4 cups chopped frozen broccoli, thawed
	1 teaspoon chopped jarred garlic, rinsed
	1 teaspoon dried basil
	1 teaspoon dried oregano
1 carbohydrate	Half a 13½-ounce can Del Monte stewed Italian-style zucchini, drained
3 carbohydrate	1½ cups Classico Basil Marinara Sauce
6 protein, 2 fat	6 ounces Tyson Grilled Chicken Strips, thawed
2 carbohydrate	1 cup roasted peppers, packed in water, drained and chopped
1 carbohydrate	One 9-ounce package frozen Bird's Eye artichoke hearts
2 protein, 2 fat	½ cup shredded skim milk mozzarella
4 fat	8 tablespoons Marie's Reduced Calorie Creamy Italian Garlic Dressing

Instructions

1 Preheat the oven to 350°F.

2 Lightly spray a nonstick skillet with olive oil cooking spray and add the broccoli, garlic, basil, and oregano. Sauté over high heat for 3 to 4 minutes.

3 In a 9 × 12-inch baking dish, layer the zucchini, packing it tightly together to make the bottom layer of the lasagna. Top with the broccoli and spread half the pasta sauce on the broccoli. Layer on the chicken, peppers, artichoke hearts, and remaining pasta sauce. Sprinkle the mozzarella on top and drizzle on the dressing. Bake 25 minutes, uncovered, or until bubbly.

New Orleans Turkey Gumbo Casserole

Diane Manteca

Prep: 5 minutes   **Yield:**   2 (4-block) servings
Cooking: 15 minutes

Block Size	Ingredients
1 carbohydrate	10 ounces mixed chopped frozen peppers
1 carbohydrate	1½ cups chopped frozen onions
	1 tablespoon chopped jarred garlic, rinsed
	1 tablespoon chili powder
	1 tablespoon cumin powder
	Kosher salt and pepper to taste
6 protein, 6½ fat	10 ounces turkey kielbasa, cut into 1-inch pieces
2 protein, 3 carbohydrate, 1½ fat	1 can Healthy Choice Gumbo Soup
3 carbohydrate	¾ cup black beans, canned and drained
	Chopped fresh parsley for garnish

Instructions

Spray a nonstick skillet, spray with olive oil cooking spray. Over high heat, sauté the peppers, onions, garlic, chili powder, cumin, salt, and pepper for 2 minutes, or until the onions are softened. Add the kielbasa and sauté 2 minutes. Add the soup and black beans, bring to a simmer, and cook 10 minutes, or until the gumbo is the desired consistency. Garnish with chopped parsley.

Calabrian Turkey "Margarita" with Chickpea and String Bean Salad

Diane Manteca

Prep: 10 minutes
Cooking: 20 minutes

Yield: 2 (4-block) servings

Block Size	Ingredients
Turkey	
2 carbohydrate	1 ounce non-steel-cut oatmeal
	1 tablespoon dried basil
	½ teaspoon kosher or sea salt
	Black pepper to taste
1 protein	¼ cup liquid egg white product
7 protein, 2 fat	7 ounces fresh turkey cutlets
2 carbohydrate	1 cup tomato sauce
Chickpea and String Bean Salad	
2 carbohydrate	½ cup canned chickpeas, drained
1 carbohydrate	1 14½-ounce can cut Italian string beans
1 carbohydrate	½ cup drained and sliced roasted peppers
4 fat	2⅔ teaspoons extra-virgin olive oil
2 fat	1 tablespoon toasted pine nuts
	1 teaspoon chopped jarred garlic, rinsed
	Salt and pepper to taste

Instructions

1 Preheat the oven to 400°F. Spray an 8 × 8-inch baking dish with olive oil cooking spray.

2 Grind the oatmeal in a food processor to the texture of bread crumbs. In a small bowl, mix the oatmeal, basil, salt, and pepper. Pour the egg product into a separate bowl. Dip the turkey cutlets first in the egg product, then in the oatmeal mixture, and place in the baking dish. Bake 15 minutes. Spread the tomato sauce on top and bake 10 minutes, or until the sauce is bubbling.

3 In a medium bowl, combine the ingredients for the chickpea and string bean salad. Season with salt and pepper. Serve the salad with the turkey cutlets.

Open-Faced Smoked Turkey Panini with Sicilian Green Bean Salad

Diane Manteca

Prep: 10 minutes
Cooking: 2 minutes

Yield: 2 (4-block) servings

Block Size	Ingredients

Turkey Panini

Block Size	Ingredients
3 carbohydrate	2 slices French Meadow bread
	2 cups baby greens or chopped romaine lettuce
6 protein	6 ounces Louis Rich fat-free hickory smoked turkey breast
1 carbohydrate	½ cup roasted peppers, drained and sliced thin
2 protein	½ cup shredded fat-free mozzarella
2 fat	1⅓ teaspoons extra-virgin olive oil

Sicilian Green Bean Salad

Block Size	Ingredients
2 carbohydrate	3 cups thawed frozen whole string beans
2 carbohydrate	⅔ cup water-packed Mandarin oranges, drained
6 fat	4 teaspoons olive oil
	Balsamic vinegar to taste
	½ cup thinly sliced red onions
	1 teaspoon dried basil
	Kosher salt and pepper to taste

Instructions

1 To make the panini, place 2 slices of the bread on a cookie sheet. Heat the broiler or toaster oven. Layer the greens or lettuce, turkey, peppers, and mozzarella on the bread and drizzle with the olive oil. Place the sandwiches under the broiler until the cheese is slightly melted, about 2 minutes.

2 In a large bowl, combine the salad ingredients. Serve with the panini.

Chicken Diablo with Oven-Roasted Vegetables

Diane Manteca

Prep: 15 minutes
Cooking: 20 minutes

Yield: 2 (4-block) servings

Block Size	Ingredients
8 protein, 2 fat	8 ounces fresh boneless chicken tenderloins
	Dijon mustard to taste
1 carbohydrate	4 cups frozen broccoli florets
1 carbohydrate	4 cups frozen cauliflower florets
1 carbohydrate	½ cup roasted peppers, drained and chopped
1 carbohydrate	1 cup frozen baby carrots
	1 tablespoon chopped jarred garlic, rinsed
	1 tablespoon dried basil
	1 tablespoon dried oregano
	1 teaspoon dried rosemary
	Kosher or sea salt to taste
	Black pepper to taste
6 fat	4 teaspoons olive oil
4 carbohydrate	1 cup dark red kidney beans, drained

Instructions

1 Preheat the oven to 400°F. Spray a 9 × 12-inch baking dish with olive oil cooking spray. Place the chicken in the dish and smear it liberally with Dijon mustard.

2 In a large mixing bowl, combine the broccoli, cauliflower, roasted peppers, carrots, garlic, basil, oregano, and rosemary and a sprinkle of salt and pepper. Drizzle with the olive oil. Spread the vegetables on a cookie sheet and spray lightly with olive oil cooking spray.

3 Roast the chicken and vegetables for 15 minutes, or until the chicken is cooked through. Toss the vegetables with the kidney beans and serve.

Autumn Chicken in Cider Sauce with Roasted Vegetables

Diane Manteca

Prep: 10 minutes
Cooking: 20 minutes

Yield: 2 (4-block) servings

Block Size	Ingredients
Roasted Vegetables	
1 carbohydrate	4 cups Green Giant frozen broccoli, carrot and cauliflower combo
	2 tablespoons chopped jarred garlic, rinsed
6 fat	4 teaspoons extra-virgin olive oil
	½ teaspoon dried thyme
	½ teaspoon dried basil
	½ teaspoon dried oregano
	Kosher salt and pepper to taste
Chicken	
	½ cup frozen chopped onions
	1 tablespoon chopped jarred garlic, rinsed
	Kosher salt and pepper to taste
8 protein, 2 fat	8 ounces fresh chicken tenderloins
1 carbohydrate	½ cup dry white wine
1 carbohydrate	⅓ cup apple cider
1 carbohydrate	⅓ cup unsweetened applesauce
	1 cup chicken stock
4 carbohydrate	2 cups Campbell's 98 percent fat-free condensed cream of celery soup

Instructions

1 To make the vegetables, preheat the oven to 450°F. Spray a cookie sheet with olive oil cooking spray. In a medium bowl, toss the vegetables, garlic, olive oil, thyme, basil, oregano, salt, and pepper. Spread the vegetables evenly on the cookie sheet and spray them lightly with olive oil cooking spray. Roast until slightly charred, about 15 minutes.

2 To make the chicken, spray a large nonstick skillet with olive oil cooking spray. Add the onions, garlic, and a sprinkle of salt and pepper and sauté over medium heat until translucent, 3 to 4 minutes. Add the chicken and cook 4 to 5 minutes, turning once to brown both sides. Add the wine, bring to a boil, and simmer 2 to 3 minutes. Add the cider, applesauce, stock, and soup and simmer 2 to 3 minutes, or until desired consistency. Taste and season with salt and pepper as desired.

Spicy Smoked Turkey and Bean Fiesta Stew

Diane Manteca

Prep: 10 minutes
Cooking: 10 minutes

Yield: 2 (4-block) servings

Block Size	Ingredients
6 fat	4 teaspoons olive oil
8 protein, 2 fat	12 ounces smoked deli turkey breast, cut into 1-inch pieces
	1 teaspoon chili powder
	1 teaspoon cumin powder
	½ teaspoon kosher salt
3½ carbohydrate	One 18.6-ounce can Campbell's Select Fiesta Vegetable Soup
2 carbohydrate	½ cup canned black beans, drained and rinsed
1½ carbohydrate	⅓ cup chickpeas, drained and rinsed
1 carbohydrate	½ cup Old El Paso Homestyle Salsa

Instructions

In a large saucepan over high heat, heat the olive oil. Add the turkey, chili powder, cumin, and salt and cook, stirring constantly, 1 or 2 minutes. Add the remaining ingredients and bring to a boil. Serve in large soup bowls.

Florentine Spinach and Ricotta Stuffed Chicken

Diane Manteca

Prep: 10 minutes
Cooking: 15 minutes

Yield: 2 (4-block) servings

Block Size

Ingredients

Chicken

	1 cup Bird's Eye chopped frozen spinach, thawed
2 carbohydrate	1 cup jarred roasted peppers, drained and finely chopped
2 protein, 2 fat	½ cup skim milk ricotta cheese
	1 teaspoon kosher salt
	½ teaspoon black pepper
6 protein, 1½ fat	6 ounces boneless skinless chicken breast, cut into two pieces
4½ fat	2⅔ teaspoons olive oil
3 carbohydrate	1½ cups Classico Basil Marinara Sauce

Vegetables

1 carbohydrate	1½ cups chopped frozen onions
1 carbohydrate	2 cups sliced zucchini
1 carbohydrate	2 cups sliced summer squash
	1 teaspoon chopped jarred garlic, rinsed
	1 teaspoon dried basil
	1 teaspoon dried oregano
	Kosher salt and pepper to taste

Instructions

1 Spray a baking dish with olive oil cooking spray and preheat the oven to 350° F. Squeeze the liquid from the spinach. In a medium bowl, combine the spinach, peppers, ricotta, ½ of the teaspoon salt, and ¼ teaspoon of the pepper. Cut a slit in the side of each piece of chicken to create a pocket. Divide the ricotta-spinach stuffing between the two chicken pockets. Place the chicken in the baking dish, drizzle the olive oil evenly on top, and sprinkle with the remaining ½ teaspoon salt and ¼ teaspoon pepper. Bake for 20 minutes, or until light golden brown. Heat the marinara sauce in the microwave or in a small saucepan over low heat.

2 While the chicken is baking, spray a nonstick skillet with olive oil cooking spray. Add the olive oil, onions, zucchini, summer squash, garlic, basil, oregano, and salt and pepper to taste and sauté over medium-high heat 5 minutes, or until just tender.

3 Divide the sautéed vegetables between 2 plates. Place the chicken on top and pour the marinara sauce over the chicken.

Steak Pizziola

Diane Manteca

Prep: 8 minutes
Cooking: 10 minutes

Yield: 2 (4-block) servings

Block Size	Ingredients
3 fat	2 teaspoons extra-virgin olive oil
1 carbohydrate	1½ cups chopped frozen onions
	1 tablespoon dried oregano
	½ teaspoon kosher salt
	½ teaspoon black pepper
	1 tablespoon chopped jarred garlic, rinsed
8 protein, 5 fat	8 ounces lean beef round steak, sliced thin
1 carbohydrate	6 sun-dried tomatoes packed in oil, drained and chopped
2 carbohydrate	1 cup Del Monte diced tomatoes with basil, oregano, and garlic, with juices
3 carbohydrate	¾ cup Progresso fava beans, drained and rinsed
1 carbohydrate	One 14½-ounce can Del Monte cut Italian green beans, drained

Instructions

In a nonstick skillet, heat the olive oil on high. Sauté the onions, oregano, salt, and pepper 1 minute, add the garlic, and sauté 1 or 2 minutes, or until the onions are softened. Push the onions to the side of the pan and add the steak. Stirring constantly, sauté 3 minutes, or until the steak begins to lose its pink color. Lower the heat to medium and add the sun-dried tomatoes, diced tomatoes, fava beans, and green beans. Stir well and cook 5 minutes, or until the mixture is hot.

Beef Bourguignonne

Diane Manteca

Prep: 8 minutes   **Yield:**   2 (4-block) servings
Cooking: 25 minutes

Block Size	Ingredients
3 fat	2 teaspoons olive oil
8 protein, 5 fat	8 ounces lean beef round sandwich steaks, cut in 1-inch slices
	Kosher or sea salt and black pepper to taste
	2 tablespoons chopped jarred garlic, rinsed
1 carbohydrate	2 cups frozen pearl onions
1 carbohydrate	2½ cups canned sliced mushrooms, drained
1 carbohydrate	1 cup canned Green Giant LaSuer baby carrots
	1 cup fat-free beef broth
4 carbohydrate	2 cups Campbell's Select 98 percent fat-free condensed cream of mushroom soup
	2 tablespoons tomato paste
	½ teaspoon dried thyme
1 carbohydrate	1½ cups Green Giant frozen cut green beans, thawed

Instructions

In a nonstick skillet over high heat, heat olive oil. Add the beef, sprinkle it with kosher or sea salt and black pepper. Sauté on both sides for 4 to 5 minutes, or until golden brown. Add the garlic, pearl onions, mushrooms, carrots, broth, soup, tomato paste, and thyme. Bring to a boil, then lower the heat to medium-low and cook for 20 minutes. Add the green beans and cook 2 more minutes, or until heated through.

Moroccan Chicken Stew

Diane Manteca

Prep: 8 minutes
Cooking: 10 minutes

Yield: 2 (4-block) servings

Block Size	Ingredients
3½ fat	2½ teaspoons extra-virgin olive oil
7 protein, 2½ fat	1½ cups Perdue Shortcuts Chicken Breast, Roasted Original, cut into 1-inch pieces
	1 tablespoon chopped jarred garlic, rinsed
	1 or 2 tablespoons curry powder (to taste)
	½ teaspoon ground cinnamon
	1 teaspoon dried cumin
	1 teaspoon kosher salt
1 carbohydrate	⅓ cup Del Monte lite apricots, drained and sliced
3 carbohydrate	¾ cup canned chickpeas, drained
2 fat, 2 carbohydrate, 1 protein	1 can Campbell's Healthy Request cream of chicken soup
1 carbohydrate	2 cups Green Giant San Francisco frozen vegetable mix

Instructions

In a large, heavy saucepan over high heat, heat the olive oil. Add the chicken, garlic, curry powder, cinnamon, cumin, and salt and sauté for 2 minutes, or until the chicken is heated through. Add the remaining ingredients and bring to a boil. Serve in large soup bowls.

Summer Chicken BBQ with Coleslaw and Grilled Vegetables

Diane Manteca

Prep: 10 minutes
Cooking: 20 minutes

Yield: 2 (4-block) servings

Block Size	Ingredients
Coleslaw	
3 carbohydrate	5 tablespoons Kraft Free ranch dressing
	½ teaspoon Dijon mustard
2 fat	4 teaspoons Hellman's light mayonnaise
	1 tablespoon cider vinegar
	½ teaspoon kosher salt
1 carbohydrate	Half a 16-ounce bag dry coleslaw mix
Vegetables	
1 carbohydrate	4 cups frozen cauliflower florets, thawed
1 carbohydrate	2 cups cherry tomatoes
1 carbohydrate	4 cups frozen broccoli florets, thawed
	2 tablespoons chopped jarred garlic, rinsed
	1 teaspoon dried oregano
	1 teaspoon dried basil
	½ teaspoon kosher salt
	¼ teaspoon black pepper
Chicken	
8 protein, 2 fat	8 ounces boneless skinless fresh chicken breast
4 fat	2⅔ teaspoons extra-virgin olive oil
	Kosher salt and pepper to taste
1 carbohydrate	2 tablespoons hickory-smoked barbecue sauce

Instructions

1 To make the coleslaw, in a large bowl, whisk the ranch dressing, Dijon mustard, mayonnaise, cider vinegar, and salt. Add the coleslaw mix, toss, and refrigerate until ready to serve.

2 Preheat the grill.

3 In a large bowl, mix the cauliflower, cherry tomatoes, broccoli, garlic, oregano, basil, salt, and pepper. Make a foil packet from heavy-duty aluminum foil. Put the vegetables in the foil packet, spray with olive oil cooking spray, toss, spray again, and seal.

4 Brush the chicken breasts with the olive oil and sprinkle with a little salt and pepper.

5 Place the vegetable packet and the chicken on the grill. Cook the chicken, turning occasionally, until done in the center, about 15 minutes. Brush the barbecue sauce on top of the chicken. Turn the vegetable packet after 5 minutes and grill until tender, about another 5 minutes.

6 Serve the chicken with the coleslaw and vegetables on the side.

Baked Greek Shrimp and Feta with Dill Cucumber Salad

Diane Manteca

Prep: 8 minutes
Cooking: 15 minutes

Yield: 2 (4-block) servings

Block Size	Ingredients
Shrimp	
2 protein, 6½ fat	½ cup crumbled Athenos reduced-fat feta cheese
6 protein, 1½ fat	9 ounces large raw shrimp, peeled and deveined
1 carbohydrate	1½ cups chopped frozen onions
3 carbohydrate	¾ cups canned red kidney beans, drained
2 carbohydrate	1 cup Del Monte canned diced tomatoes with basil, garlic, and oregano, with juices
	1 tablespoon chopped jarred garlic, rinsed
	1 tablespoon dried oregano
Cucumber Salad	
2 carbohydrate	3 medium cucumbers, peeled and sliced thin
	1 tablespoon lemon juice or red wine vinegar
	½ teaspoon dried dill
	½ teaspoon kosher salt
	¼ teaspoon black pepper
	Lettuce leaves

Instructions

1 Preheat the oven to 400° F.

2 In a 9 × 9-inch casserole or baking dish, combine the feta, shrimp, onions, kidney beans, tomatoes, garlic, and oregano and mix well. Bake 15 minutes, or until the shrimp is curled and pink.

3 In a medium bowl, combine the cucumber salad ingredients and spray with olive oil cooking spray. Serve the salad on lettuce leaves next to the shrimp.

Grilled Napoli Pizzas with Spinach and Mushrooms and Turkey Bacon Salad

Diane Manteca

Prep: 8 minutes
Cooking: 10 minutes

Yield: 2 (4-block) servings

Block Size	Ingredients
Pizzas	
4 carbohydrate	Two 8-inch flour tortillas
4 protein	4 ounces shredded fat-free mozzarella cheese
	1 teaspoon dried oregano
	½ teaspoon kosher salt
	¼ teaspoon black pepper
1 carbohydrate	2 ripe tomatoes, sliced
1½ carbohydrate	¾ cup thinly sliced roasted red peppers, drained
Salad	
½ carbohydrate	2 cups sliced fresh mushrooms
	5 cups fresh baby spinach
2 protein, 5 fat	6 slices cooked turkey bacon, chopped
2 protein	2 ounces nonfat cheese, shredded
3 fat	2 teaspoons extra-virgin olive oil
	1 tablespoon red wine vinegar
	½ teaspoon kosher salt
	¼ teaspoon black pepper
1 carbohydrate	1 cup sliced fresh strawberries

Instructions

1 Prepare the pizzas on a cutting board or other surface that can be transferred to a grill. Spray both sides of the tortillas with olive oil cooking spray. Top each with the mozzarella, oregano, salt, and pepper. Layer the tomatoes and roasted peppers evenly on top. Spray the pizzas lightly with olive oil cooking spray. Carefully slide the pizzas onto the hot grill. Put the grill cover down and cook 5 minutes, or until the cheese is melted.

2 In a large bowl, mix all the salad ingredients together. Serve the salad with the pizza and serve the strawberries for dessert.

Note: The pizza can also be baked on a cookie sheet at 400°F. Bake until the cheese is melted and bubbly, 8 to10 minutes.

Italian Frittata with Tuscan White Bean Soup

Diane Manteca

Prep: 10 minutes
Cooking: 10 minutes

Yield: 2 (4-block) servings

Block Size	Ingredients
5 fat	3⅓ teaspoons light olive oil
1 carbohydrate	1½ cups chopped frozen onions
	2 scallions (green onions), chopped
1 carbohydrate	One 9-ounce package frozen Bird's Eye artichoke hearts, thawed
	1 cup chopped frozen spinach, thawed and squeezed
2 carbohydrate	1 cup chopped roasted red peppers, drained
	½ teaspoon kosher salt
	¼ teaspoon black pepper
6 protein	1½ cups liquid egg white product
2 protein, 3 fat	7 tablespoons grated imported low-fat Parmesan cheese

Soup

Block Size	Ingredients
3 carbohydrate	3 cups Healthy Choice Mediterranean pasta and bean soup
1 carbohydrate	½ cup canned cannellini beans, drained
	½ cup chicken stock
	¼ teaspoon dry rosemary, crumbled
	Kosher salt and pepper to taste

Instructions

1 To make the frittata, in a nonstick sauté pan over medium heat, heat the olive oil. Add the onions, scallion (green onions), artichoke hearts, spinach, red peppers, salt, and pepper and sauté 2 minutes. Add the egg product and stir them around in the pan. Lower the heat to medium-low and cook, undisturbed, 3 or 4 minutes. Sprinkle with the cheese. Cover the pan and cook 1 or 2 minutes, or until the eggs are set. Slide the frittata out of the pan and cut it in half.

2 To make the soup, in a medium saucepan over medium heat, bring the pasta and bean soup to a boil. Add the beans, stock, and rosemary and heat through. Season with salt and pepper to taste.

3 Serve the frittata on plates with the soup in bowls on the side.

Hungarian Beef Goulash

Diane Manteca

Prep: 10 minutes   **Yield:**   2 (4-block) servings
Cooking: 15 minutes

Block Size	Ingredients
3 fat	2 teaspoons extra-virgin olive oil
6 protein, 5 fat	6 ounces lean beef round steak, sliced thin
	1 teaspoon caraway seeds
	1 teaspoon paprika
	1 teaspoon kosher salt
	½ teaspoon black pepper
½ carbohydrate	¾ cups chopped frozen onions
½ carbohydrate	2 cups sliced canned mushrooms, drained
2 carbohydrate	1 cup Campbell's Select 98 percent fat-free mushroom soup
2 carbohydrate	1 cup canned Del Monte diced tomatoes, with juices
1 carbohydrate	2 cups thawed frozen cut string beans
	1 tablespoon chopped jarred garlic, rinsed
2 protein, 2 carbohydrate	1 cup plain nonfat yogurt

Instructions

1 In a large, heavy saucepan over high heat, heat the olive oil. Add the beef, caraway seeds, paprika, salt, and pepper and sauté 5 minutes, or until the beef loses its pink color. Add the onions and mushrooms and sauté 3 minutes. Lower the heat to medium and add the soup, tomatoes, string beans, and garlic. Bring the mixture to a boil and simmer 10 minutes.

2 In a small bowl, whisk the yogurt until it reaches a creamy consistency. Stir the yogurt into the goulash and turn off the heat. Serve in large bowls.

Chicken Tetrazzini

Diane Manteca

Prep: 8 minutes
Cooking: 15 minutes

Yield: 2 (4-block) servings

Block Size	Ingredients
4½ fat	1 tablespoon extra-virgin olive oil
1 carbohydrate	2½ cups canned asparagus
1 carbohydrate	2½ cups sliced canned mushrooms, drained
	1 tablespoon chopped jarred garlic, rinsed
	1 teaspoon dried basil
	1 teaspoon dried oregano
	1 teaspoon kosher salt
	¼ teaspoon black pepper
6 protein, 1½ fat	6 ounces chicken tenderloins
1 carbohydrate	½ cup dry white wine
4 carbohydrate	2 cups Campbell's Select 98 percent fat-free condensed cream of mushroom soup
2 protein, 2 fat	4 tablespoon grated imported low-fat Parmesan cheese
1 carbohydrate	⅓ cup hot cooked long-grain white rice

Instructions

In a heavy nonstick sauté pan over high heat, heat the olive oil. Add the asparagus, mushrooms, garlic, basil, oregano, salt, and pepper and cook 1 minute. Add the chicken and white wine and cook 2 minutes, or until the chicken is cooked through. Add the soup, bring the mixture to a quick boil, and turn off the heat. Taste for seasoning and stir in the Parmesan cheese. Serve over the rice.

DESSERTS

Ricotta Candita

Diane Manteca

Prep: 10 minutes   **Yield:**   4 (1-block) servings

Block Size	Ingredients
2 protein, 2 fat	½ cup skim milk ricotta cheese
2 carbohydrate, 2 protein	1 cup nonfat plain yogurt
1 carbohydrate	2 teaspoons fructose powder
	2 tablespoons dark rum
	2 tablespoons decaffeinated espresso or
	dark roast brewed coffee
1 carbohydrate	1 cup fresh raspberries
2 fat	4 teaspoons chopped toasted almonds

Instructions

In a medium bowl, blend the ricotta and yogurt until smooth. Add the fructose, rum, and espresso or coffee. Blend well. Divide into 4 elegant bowls or wineglasses and top with the raspberries and almonds.

Baked Stuffed Peaches with Yogurt-Cinnamon Sauce

Diane Manteca

Prep: 8 minutes   **Yield:**   4 (1-block) desserts
Cooking: 25 minutes

Block Size	Ingredients
2 carbohydrate	2 fresh, ripe peaches, cut in half, pit removed
	Zest of 1 orange
2 protein, 1 fat	½ cup low-fat, small curd cottage cheese
2 protein, 2 carbohydrate	1 cup nonfat plain yogurt
	1 tablespoon vanilla
	1 teaspoon cinnamon
	Dash of nutmeg
3 fat	12 toasted cashews, roughly chopped

Instructions

1 Preheat the oven to 350°F.

2 Place the peaches in a small baking dish. Divide the orange zest among the 4 peach halves, filling the cavity. Bake 25 minutes, or until the peaches are just cooked through.

3 In a blender, combine the cottage cheese, yogurt, vanilla, cinnamon, and nutmeg and blend until smooth. Divide the sauce onto 4 dessert plates and place the peaches and any juices on top. Garnish with the toasted cashews.

Tiramisu

Diane Manteca

Prep: 10 minutes   **Yield:** 4 (1-block) servings

Block Size	Ingredients
2⅔ carbohydrate	2 full sheets Honey Maid low-fat cinnamon graham crackers (2 crackers per sheet)
2 protein	½ cup liquid egg white product*
2 protein	½ cup fat-free ricotta cheese
	1 tablespoon brandy
	2 tablespoons decaffeinated brewed espresso or dark roast coffee
1⅓ carbohydrate	2½ teaspoons fructose powder
	2 tablespoons unsweetened cocoa
4 fat	8 teaspoons toasted slivered almonds

Instructions

1 Break the sheets of crackers in half so that you have 4 pieces.

2 In a medium bowl, whip the egg product until fluffy with an electric mixer. In a separate large bowl, whisk the ricotta, brandy, espresso or coffee, and fructose until fluffy. Very carefully fold in the egg.

3 Place one cracker on each of 4 dessert plates. Divide the ricotta mixture on top of the 4 crackers. Dust with the cocoa. Top with the almonds, or arrange them around the plates.

Note: Egg product has been pasteurized and homogenized.

Berries Zabaglione

Diane Manteca

Prep: 10 minutes

Yield: 4 (1-block) servings

Block Size	Ingredients
1 carbohydrate	1 cup thinly sliced fresh strawberries
2 carbohydrate	1 cup fresh blueberries
4 protein	1 cup liquid egg white product*
1 carbohydrate	2 teaspoons fructose powder
	1 teaspoon vanilla
	2 tablespoons Marsala (or other sweet) wine
4 fat	8 teaspoons toasted slivered almonds

Instructions

Combine the strawberries and blueberries in a small Pyrex or other ovenproof baking dish. In a medium bowl, combine the egg product, fructose, vanilla, and Marsala wine and whip until fluffy with an electric mixer. Pour the mixture over the berries. Place the dish under the broiler for 2 minutes, or until light golden brown. Top with the almonds and serve immediately.

Note: Egg product has been pasteurized and homogenized.

9

Slow Cooking in the Zone

In the last chapter, we showed how quickly you can put together a Zone meal using convenience foods. In this chapter, we're going to slow it down a bit. Meal preparation will still be quick, but your delicious Zone dinner will cook slowly throughout the day. Rachel Albert Matesz wrote these tips.

Slow cooking might sound old-fashioned—as evidenced by Minute Rice, frozen dinners, instant soup, and microwave ovens—but before you dismiss the idea, take another look. Slow cookers are the ideal appliance for busy people, single people, married people, and those with kids or without.

Slow cookers are versatile, convenient, portable, easy to use, and energy efficient. A slow cooker uses less electricity than a 75 to 100 watt lightbulb and eats up less energy than an electric oven or range. The low temperature won't overheat your kitchen, even during the hottest months of the year.

Slow cookers allow you to start foods and leave them unattended while you do laundry, chase after the kids, run errands, work, play, or tend the yard. If you don't want to fire up the oven on a hot day, if you're short on burners, if find your oven on the fritz, if your kitchen is being remodeled, or if you want homemade hot cereal in a motel room, you can rely on a slow cooker.

A slow cooker can help tenderize lean or tough cuts of meat while simultaneously softening hardy root vegetables. Besides brewing up soup, stew, and chili, your slow cooker can cook main dishes such as roast chicken, chicken parts, turkey breast, beef, bison, pork, lamb, roasts, fillets, cubes, and chops. You can slowly simmer breakfast porridge while you sleep; roast vegetables, bake apples, or poach pears while you pick up the kids; or cook a casserole while you clean the house.

You no longer need to worry about pots running dry and food burning. Stirring is rarely required. Cooking times are also more flexible, whereas more exact cooking times are required for direct heat cooking (on the grill, in the oven, or on the stove). The indirect and low heat of a slow cooker will give you a larger margin for error: 30 minutes more or less won't ruin a dish.

To take food to a picnic or potluck, cook the dish at home, wrap the filled slow cooker and lid in two layers of aluminum foil and five or six layers of newspaper, secure the bundle with heavy duty tape, and place the cooker upright in a box. As long as you keep it upright, your dish will be company-ready when you arrive, at which point you can plug it in and warm the contents on LOW.

WHAT EXACTLY IS A SLOW COOKER?

A slow cooker consists of a glazed, usually stoneware, ceramic, or porcelain, insert pot or crock (some are removable, some aren't) and a see-through heavy glass lid. Some models now come with plastic lids. The crockery pot nests inside a metal housing that contains low-wattage, wrap-around electric heating coils, which surround the food and cooking vessel with continuous, even, and indirect heat. A slow cooker features two temperature settings: LOW (200°F) and HIGH (300°F).

HOW DOES A SLOW COOKER WORK?

While conventional cooking requires that you bring a pot to boil, then reduce the heat, slow cookers work in reverse. Food in a slow cooker starts cooking at a low temperature and gradually becomes hotter as the cooking time progresses. The rising temperature, long cooking time, and a tight-fitting lid generate heat, seal in moisture, and kill bacteria.

When you turn on a slow cooker, the elements contained inside the double-walled metal housing heat up and warm the air trapped between the two metal walls. When the metal walls get hot, they transfer their heat to the stoneware crock, and then to the food inside. Since the heating elements never come in direct contact with the crockery insert, you'll never have hot spots, and your food will rarely require stirring.

SHOPPING FOR A SLOW COOKER

The terms slow cooker, Crock Pot®, and crockery cooker all refer to the same basic appliance. Slow cooker and crockery cooker are generic terms. Crock Pot® is a registered trademark of Rival, not a generic term. Rival is the grandfather of slow cookers. Hamilton Beach is the second leading manufacturer of slow cookers.

Some manufacturers call their multipurpose cookers "slow cookers." These appliances warm foods, boil, steam, stew, roast, and fry. Some look like electric deep-dish skillets with lids; others resemble deep-fat fryers. These units usually come with a removable metal pot that sits directly above a coiled heating element, which cycles on and off. Because these units cook with direct heat, they heat up more quickly, more moisture is lost through evaporation, and foods are apt to stick and burn unless you stir frequently. This means that you can't leave them unattended, and that foods left for seven or eight hours are apt to overcook. Pseudo-slow cookers feature variable, numbered dial settings that range from warming to deep-frying temperatures, as opposed to the LOW and HIGH settings on a true slow cooker. These appliances require different cooking times and methods. For the best results with the recipes contained in this book, we recommend that you purchase a true slow cooker.

WHAT SIZE AND SHAPE SHOULD I BUY?

Today's modern slow cookers come in an assortment of sizes, ranging from 1- to 7 quart capacity models. A slow cooker is designed to work best when filled at least one-half and not more than three-quarters full. Select a size that accommodates your family's needs.

The smallest units (1- to 1½-quart size) are often sold as Crockettes and have only two settings, on and off. They are ideal for heating party dips or making hot cereal for one or two people. The 3½- and 4-quart models are the most versatile. Larger units are best for big families or entertaining. If you plan to do a lot of slow cooking, you may want to buy two different sizes.

Slow cookers are sold in most department stores, general stores, and discount merchandise outlets. You can also buy them online. Sometimes you'll find them on sale or at thrift stores or garage sales. Maybe someone you know has a slow cooker in the attic or basement that has never been used and needs a new home. Make calls and inquire with friends and family.

Slow cookers come in round and oval shapes. Round cookers are ideal for soup, stew, sauces, oatmeal, and casseroles. The oval design is perfect for roasting whole chickens, turkey breasts, and roasts that would not ordinarily fit into a round cooker, although it may be used to cook other entrées. Rival makes a 5-quart slow cooker with a divided cooking compartment that allows you to cook two dishes at the same time—say, a pork roast in the large compartment and roasted vegetables in the smaller compartment—without flavor mixing.

Slow cookers with removable ceramic inserts are easier to clean than one-piece units. Glass lids are generally more durable and less apt to absorb flavors or aromas than plastic lids. If you plan to take your slow cooker to parties or community events, look for a slow cooker with a lid latch and insulated carrying case. Both Rival and Hamilton Beach feature these models, with carrying cases sold separately.

CARING FOR YOUR SLOW COOKER

- Read the manufacturer's instruction booklet that comes with your slow cooker for safety tips and usage guidelines.

- Do not heat the stoneware crockery insert on a stove or cook top. Removable stoneware inserts are oven- and microwave-proof. One-piece slow cookers are not.

- Do not use a slow cooker outdoors.

- Avoid sudden temperature changes. Do not place a hot slow cooker in the refrigerator or freezer and avoid adding cold foods or cold water to a hot cooker. Dramatic changes in temperature can cause cracking or breakage.

- Avoid running water over a hot cooking container or cover. Allow it to cool thoroughly.

- Do not preheat an empty slow cooker container. Turn it on after adding food or liquids.

- Wash your slow cooker as soon as possible after emptying and unplugging.

- Do not use harsh cleaning agents or abrasive scouring pads to clean your slow cooker. Use soap, warm water, and a sponge or dishcloth, and then dry with a soft cloth.

- Removable stoneware inserts and lids can be safely washed in a dishwasher or by hand. Plastic lids should be placed in the top of your dishwasher to avoid warping. The outside case may be cleaned with a dishcloth and warm, soapy water.

- The inside of the base of your slow cooker should be wiped clean after use to remove any particles of food or traces of oil.

- Do not immerse one-piece units or their cords in water.

- Do not use a slow cooker container or lid that is chipped, cracked, or deeply scratched.

- Do not use your slow cooker to store foods. Always transfer cooked foods to new containers.

- Do not use a slow cooker to defrost frozen foods or to warm previously cooked foods.

- Avoid touching the sides or lid of a slow cooker that is turned on. They can get extremely hot.

TIPS FOR SLOW COOKING SUCCESS

- Thaw frozen foods before adding them to your slow cooker.

- Keep all perishable foods in the refrigerator until you are ready to cook them. If you plan to chop vegetables or meats the night before, store them in separate containers in the refrigerator.

- Remove the skin from poultry and trim away visible fat from meat and poultry before cooking.

- Avoid removing the lid during cooking, unless specified in a recipe. Only remove the lid to stir (if called for) or to check for doneness. It can take 15 to 20 minutes for a slow cooker to regain lost heat after the lid has been removed.

- Unless indicated, place tubers and root vegetables in the bottom of the slow cooker, with meats, seasonings, and quick-cooking vegetables or fruits on top.

- If a recipe calls for browning, brown the meat in a skillet on top of the stove, then add it to the cooker. A portion of the liquid from the recipe may be added to the skillet to "deglaze" and gather food particles that have settled in the bottom of the sauté pan.

- When cooking at high altitudes (above 3,500 feet), it may be necessary to increase the cooking time.

- If a recipe calls for arrowroot or cornstarch to thicken a sauce, add it at the end of cooking, raise heat to HIGH, and cook for 15 to 45 minutes more to thicken. Or, transfer the liquids to a saucepan on top of the stove; bring to boil, reduce the heat, and simmer until smooth and thick.

- Dairy products should be added at the end of slow cooking, if at all.

- Most slow cooker recipes require larger amounts of herbs and spices than conventional recipes. In some cases, it is helpful to add additional herbs near the end of cooking to enhance the flavors. Whole spices become very intense in flavor if left in the pot the whole time.

- If you plan to sauté or brown foods before adding them to the pot, do this right before adding them to the cooker and turning it on. Never partially cook meat ahead of time and plan to finish cooking later.

THE HIGHS AND LOWS OF SLOW COOKING

Most foods turn out best cooked on LOW, although some recipes include the option of cooking on LOW or HIGH. It is best to use the LOW setting when you leave foods cooking unattended. The HIGH setting is best reserved for times when you will be at home to supervise the cooking. If you want to cook food faster, you can start it on LOW, then turn the dial to HIGH during the last one or two hours of cooking, or cook the food on HIGH for the entire cooking time, if the recipe lists that as an option. One hour on HIGH is equivalent to two hours on LOW.

MODIFYING YOUR FAVORITE RECIPES

Slow cooker recipes ordinarily call for less liquid than do conventional recipes. The reason: low heat and long cooking produce and retain more moisture. Since liquids do not boil away, you do not need to add as much liquid.

The majority of slow cooker recipes take 6 to 10 hours to cook. Until you are familiar with slow cooker cooking times, it is wise to follow recipes or model what you make on someone else's slow cooker recipes. If you are unsure about the doneness of a food, you can test it with an instant-read or meat thermometer, inserted into the thickest part of a roast, away from the bone, or cut into a piece of meat or cubed poultry.

SLOW-COOKING RECIPES

Chicken Breasts in Sun-Dried Tomato Sauce

Rachel Albert-Matesz

Prep: 20 minutes   **Yield:**   4 (4-block) servings
Cooking: 4 to 5½ hours

Start this chicken dish cooking in a slow cooker before you leave home to run errands, or leave it to cook while you do laundry or yard work.

Block Size	Ingredients
Chicken	
16 protein	4 small (4 ounce) boneless chicken breast halves, skin removed
1 carbohydrate	12 sun-dried tomato halves, quartered
1 carbohydrate	1½ cups onion, cut into thin half-moons
½ carbohydrate	2 cups thinly sliced mushrooms
1 carbohydrate	½ cup dry white wine
	3 garlic cloves, coarsely chopped
	½ teaspoon ground black pepper
	1 tablespoon herbes de Provence **or** Italian herb blend
2 carbohydrate	8 teaspoons cornstarch **or** arrowroot
1 carbohydrate	¼ cup apple cider
6 fat	2 tablespoons pine nuts
Fruit	
3 carbohydrate	¾ cup thawed frozen pitted unsweetened "sweet" cherries

4 carbohydrate	4 peaches, halved, pitted, and sliced **or**
	3 cups thawed frozen sliced, unsweetened
	peaches
	¼ teaspoon ground cinnamon
	1 teaspoon pure vanilla extract

Vegetables

2½ carbohydrate	One 16-ounce bag frozen Bird's Eye
	broccoli, cauliflower, carrots, and
	water chestnuts
	2 tablespoon organic red wine vinegar **or**
	apple cider vinegar
	2 teaspoons dry mustard plus 2 tablespoons
	water
10 fat	1 tablespoon plus ⅛ teaspoon extra-virgin
	olive oil

Instructions

1 To make the chicken, layer the chicken, tomatoes, onion, mushrooms, wine, garlic, pepper, and herbs in a 3½-quart slow cooker. Cover and cook on LOW for 4 to 5 hours.

2 Dissolve the cornstarch in the cider, add it to the slow cooker, cover, and cook on HIGH for 15 to 20 minutes, or until the sauce has thickened.

3 To make the fruit, combine the fruit, cinnamon, and vanilla. Toss, then divide among 4 serving bowls.

4 To make the vegetables, bring ½ cup water to a boil in a 1½-quart saucepan. Add the frozen vegetables, cover, and lower the heat to medium. Simmer 8 to 10 minutes, or until tender, stirring occasionally. Drain and transfer to 4 small salad plates. In a small bowl, whisk the vinegar, mustard, and oil. Drizzle the dressing over the vegetables.

5 Transfer the hot chicken and sauce to 4 shallow serving bowls. Garnish with the pine nuts and serve immediately with vegetables. Serve the fruit for dessert.

Chicken, Chickpea, and Squash Goulash with Sautéed Cabbage and Caraway

Rachel Albert-Matesz

Prep: 25 minutes   **Yield:**   4 (4-block) meals
Cooking: 6 to 8 hours

This stew has it all—sweet, sour, salty, and spicy flavors. For the sautéed cabbage, I made a few modifications to a steam-sauté recipe found in Pam Anderson's *How to Cook Without a Book,* a guide to mastering basic cooking techniques, then exploring countless variations.

Block Size	Ingredients
Goulash	
1 carbohydrate	1½ cups onion, cut into half-moon
4 carbohydrate	1 cup drained, unsalted chickpeas
16 protein	1 pound boneless skinless chicken thighs
1 carbohydrate	1 cup Eden or Cascadian Farms sauerkraut, drained
4 carbohydrate	One 10-ounce package Cascadian Farm thawed frozen organic winter squash
	1 bay leaf
	1 tablespoon hot or mild paprika
	⅛ teaspoon ground black pepper
	⅓ cup chicken stock, or as needed to moisten
1½ carbohydrate	2 tablespoons arrowroot starch
	3 tablespoons cold filtered water **or** chicken stock
8 fat	¼ cup sesame tahini
	½ teaspoon dried dill
	¼ cup minced fresh parsley **or** chives

Cabbage

	⅓ cup filtered water **or** low-sodium chicken stock or broth
8 fat	2⅔ teaspoons olive oil
	½ teaspoon sea salt (optional)
1 carbohydrate	1½ cups finely minced onion
3 carbohydrate	12 cups shredded cabbage, may be red or red and green
	2 garlic cloves, minced
	½ teaspoon ground caraway seeds

Instructions

1 Layer the onion, chickpeas, chicken, sauerkraut, squash, bay leaf, paprika, pepper, and stock in 3½- to 5-quart slow cooker. Cover and cook on LOW 6 to 8 hours.

2 About 20 minutes before serving, assemble the thickener. In a small bowl, stir the starch into the cold water or stock. Stir in the tahini and dill. Add the mixture to the cooker, cover, and turn to HIGH, stirring occasionally, until thick, about 15 minutes. Turn off the heat.

3 To make the cabbage, in a large Dutch oven or skillet, combine the water or stock, oil, salt, onion, cabbage, garlic, and caraway. Cover and bring to boil over medium-high heat. Steam until vegetables are just tender, about 10 minutes. Uncover and cook 1 to 2 minutes, or until the liquid evaporates.

4 Serve the goulash in 4 large, shallow soup bowls and garnish with the parsley or chives. Place the cabbage on 4 small salad plates and serve.

Cornish Game Hens with Salsa and Jicama, Orange, and Avocado Salad

Rachel Albert-Matesz

Prep: 20 minutes   **Yield:**   4 (4-block) servings
Cooking: 5 to 5½ hours

Experiment with different flavored salsas—mild or spicy, savory or fruity. I added avocados to a jicama and orange salad found in Mark Bittman's award-winning *How to Cook Everything.*

Block Size	Ingredients
Cornish Game Hens	
16 protein	2 Cornish game hens, thawed if frozen and cut in half
	½ teaspoon sea salt (optional)
	½ teaspoon lemon pepper
	2 garlic cloves, halved
	2 bay leaves
Jicama-Orange-Avocado Salad	
2 carbohydrate	4 cups jicama, peeled and cut into ¼-inch cubes
1 carbohydrate	⅓ cup freshly squeezed orange juice
1 carbohydrate	Juice of 1 lime
	Sea salt to taste
4 carbohydrate	2 oranges, peeled, seeded, tough parts removed
16 fat	1 cup peeled, pitted, ripe avocado, cubed
	2 tablespoons minced cilantro or fresh basil leaves
¾ carbohydrate	7½ cups romaine lettuce, washed and spun dry

1 carbohydrate	1 cup shredded carrot
¼ carbohydrate	½ cup thinly sliced celery ribs and leaves
6 carbohydrate	3 cups salsa (mild or spicy)

Instructions

1 Rinse the game hens inside and out and pat them dry. If giblets are present, rinse, cook them with the hens, and reserve them for use in another meal. Sprinkle the hens with salt and pepper. Stuff a garlic half and a bay leaf in the cavity of each hen and place in a 3½- to 4-quart slow cooker. Cover and cook on LOW for 5 to 5½ hours or HIGH for about 2½ hours, or until the hens are tender and the juices run clear when pricked with a fork.

2 To make the jicama-orange-avocado salad, in a large bowl, toss the jicama with the orange juice, lime juice, and salt. Marinate the mixture for up to 3 hours. Add the oranges, avocado, and cilantro or basil and toss to coat.

3 To serve, divide the lettuce, carrot, and celery among 4 large dinner plates. Remove the skin from the hens. Arrange one game hen half on each salad plate. Top with salsa and serve the jicama-orange-avocado salad on the side.

Lentil, Walnut, and Chicken Chili with Salad and Guacamole

Rachel Albert-Matesz

Prep: 20 minutes   **Yield:**   4 (4-block) servings
Cooking: 5 to 7 hours

Lentils, walnuts, and chicken team up to make a hearty and satisfying meal served with salad and fruit. Keep your kitchen stocked with the basics and you can assemble this in record time.

Block Size	Ingredients
Chili	
2 carbohydrate	3 cups onions, cut in half-moons
	½ teaspoon sea salt **or** 1 tablespoon tamari soy sauce
	1 bay leaf
	1½ tablespoons chili powder
	1 teaspoon ground cumin
	¼ to ½ teaspoon ground chipotle (smoked dried jalapeño pepper) **or** hot sauce
2 carbohydrate	2 cups chopped, canned no-salt-added tomatoes with juices
8 carbohydrate	2 cups canned no-salt-added lentils, cooked and drained
16 protein	24 ounces ground chicken breast
6 fat	18 walnut halves, coarsely chopped
	3 garlic cloves, minced

Salad

½ carbohydrate	5 cups spring salad mix **or** baby greens mix
1 carbohydrate	1 cup shredded carrot
½ carbohydrate	1 cup minced celery
10 fat	⅔ cup guacamole

Dessert

| 2 carbohydrate | 2 cups fresh strawberries **or** 2 plums, halved |

Instructions

1 Layer the chili ingredients, in the order listed, in 3½- to 4-quart slow cooker. Cover and cook on LOW for 5 to 7 hours. Remove the bay leaf before serving.

2 Serve the chili in shallow bowls. Divide the salad vegetables among 4 salad plates and top with the guacamole. Serve the fruit for dessert.

Variations

• Replace chicken with lean ground turkey.

• Layer the chili ingredients in a saucepan on top of the stove. Add ½ cup chicken or beef stock, cover, and bring to a boil over medium-high heat. Lower the heat to medium-low and simmer 2 hours, or until tender and juicy, stirring occasionally to prevent burning. If using a gas stove, slip a heat deflector under the pot before reducing the heat.

Kidney Bean, Walnut, and Turkey Chili with Salad and Sweet Corn

Rachel Albert-Matesz

Prep: 20 minutes   **Yield:**   4 (4-block) servings
Cooking: 5 to 7 hours

Start this stew in a slow cooker just before you leave the house to run errands, so it's ready for supper when you arrive home, or simmer it on top of the stove while you toss a salad in the evening.

Block Size	Ingredients
Chili	
2 carbohydrate	3 cups onions, cut in half-moons
	3 garlic cloves, minced
	1 bay leaf
	1½ tablespoons chili powder
	1 teaspoon ground cumin
	¼ to ½ teaspoon ground chipotle (smoked dried jalapeño pepper) **or** hot sauce
2 carbohydrate	2 cups chopped, canned no salt tomatoes with their juices
	½ teaspoon sea salt **or** 1 tablespoon tamari soy sauce
8 carbohydrate	2 cups canned no-salt added kidney beans, cooked and drained
16 protein	24 ounces lean ground turkey
6 fat	18 walnut halves, coarsely chopped

Salad

⅔ carbohydrate	7 cups spring salad mix **or** baby greens mix
⅓ carbohydrate	⅔ cup thinly sliced celery hearts
10 fat	⅔ cup guacamole

Corn

	⅛ cup filtered water
3 carbohydrate	1 ear sweet corn, cut into 4 pieces

Instructions

1 Layer the chili ingredients, in the order listed, in a 3½- to 4-quart slow cooker. Cover and cook on LOW for 5 to 7 hours.

2 Divide the salad greens and celery among 4 large dinner plates and top with the guacamole.

3 Add water to a small saucepan and arrange the sweet corn pieces in the bottom. Cover and bring to boil over medium-high heat, then lower the heat to medium and steam for 5 to 8 minutes, or until tender.

4 Transfer the corn to serving plates. Divide the chili into 4 large soup bowls and serve immediately.

Variations

- Replace the corn with 3 plums or 9 small apricots, washed, halved, and served for dessert.

- Layer the chili ingredients in a saucepan on top of the stove. Add ½ cup chicken or beef stock, cover, and bring to a boil over medium-high heat. Lower the heat to medium-low and simmer 2 hours, or until tender and juicy, stirring occasionally to prevent burning. If using a gas stove, slip a heat deflector under the pot before reducing the heat.

Turkey Sausage and Black Bean Chili with Fruit Salad

Rachel Albert-Matesz

Prep: 20 minutes   **Yield:**   4 (4-block) servings
Cooking: 2½ to 6 hours

This chili is a takeoff on one found in Mable Hoffman's *Healthy Crockery Cooking.* Start it just before you leave for work in the morning or on a lazy Sunday afternoon. Make enough to ensure leftovers that you can transport to work in a thermos the next day or freeze for a later date.

Block Size	Ingredients
Chili	
16 protein	16 ounces lean turkey **or** chicken breakfast sausage links, cut into 1-inch pieces
2 carbohydrate	One 14½-ounce can Eden no-salt-added diced whole tomatoes, with juices
1 carbohydrate	1½ cups finely diced onion
	2 small garlic cloves, minced or crushed
	1 tablespoon chili powder (mild or hot)
	¼ teaspoon ground chipotle (smoked dried jalapeño)
	1 bay leaf
5 carbohydrate	One 15-ounce can Eden organic black beans, drained
	1 tablespoon tamari soy sauce **or** dark miso
	¼ cup chopped cilantro (garnish)
8 fat	½ cup guacamole **or** mashed avocado with hot sauce

Fruit salad

4 carbohydrate	1⅓ cups cubed fresh or frozen mango chunks
2 carbohydrate	2 kiwi fruit, peeled, quartered, and cut into bite-size chunks
1½ carbohydrate	¾ cup seedless red grapes
	¼ teaspoon ground cinnamon
½ carbohydrate	Juice of ½ lime
	½ teaspoon pure vanilla extract
8 fat	Scant 3 tablespoons sunflower seeds

Instructions

1 Combine the sausage, tomatoes, onion, garlic, chili powder, chipotle, bay leaf, and beans in a 3½- to 4-quart slow cooker. Stir, cover, and cook on LOW for 5 to 6 hours or HIGH for 2½ to 3 hours, or until the onions are tender. Remove the bay leaf.

2 Thirty minutes before serving, thaw the frozen mangoes at room temperature. In a medium bowl, toss the mango, kiwi, and grapes. Sprinkle with the cinnamon, lime juice, and vanilla and toss to coat. Divide among 4 small bowls and garnish with the sunflower seeds.

3 Add the tamari to the chili, or dissolve the miso in ½ cup of hot chili, then add it back to the cooker, and stir. Divide chili among 4 soup bowls. Garnish with the cilantro, top with the guacamole, and serve. Serve the fruit salad for dessert.

Variations

Replace black beans with kidney beans or small red beans.

Roasted Turkey Breast in Spicy Mustard Sauce

Rachel Albert-Matesz

Prep: 15 minutes
Cooking: 5 to 6 hours

Yield: 12 servings (4 protein +
1 fat block per serving)

A 4-pound bone-in turkey breast will usually yield 2 quarts of cooked meat, about 3 pounds or twelve 4-ounce servings. Serve this a few days in a row and freeze extra portions in 4-, 8-, 12-, or 16-ounce amounts, so you can defrost and add them to main dish salads in mere minutes. Transfer frozen portions to the refrigerator the day before you want them so they'll be thawed in time.

Block Size	Ingredients
48 protein	4- to 4½-pound bone-in turkey breast, completely thawed if frozen, skin removed, rinsed, and patted dry
2 carbohydrate	⅔ cup apple cider **or** apple juice
12 fat	4 teaspoons extra-virgin olive oil
	2 tablespoons white mustard (True Natural Taste Red Chiles & Garlic or Smoked Green Chiles) **or** your favorite herb- or spice-infused prepared mustard
	3 cloves garlic, minced or pressed
	2 tablespoons tamari soy sauce **or** 1 teaspoon sea salt
	½ teaspoon ground red or black pepper
1 carbohydrate	4 teaspoons arrowroot starch
	3 tablespoons cold water

Instructions

1 Lightly oil a 3½- to 6-quart slow cooker. Place the turkey breast in the slow cooker.

2 In a small bowl, combine the apple cider or apple juice, olive oil, mustard, garlic, tamari or sea salt, and pepper. Whisk and pour over the turkey. Cover and cook on LOW 5 to 6 hours or HIGH for 2½ to 3 hours, or until tender and an instant-read thermometer inserted into the thickest part of the breast (away from the bone) registers 160 to 170°F, or a pop-up thermometer pops up (if one was inserted by the packager of the turkey breast).

3 Transfer the turkey breast to a meat-designated cutting board and cool 15 minutes. Transfer the cooking liquid to a small saucepan and simmer, uncovered, 15 to 20 minutes, or until reduced to about ⅔ cup. In a small bowl, dissolve the arrowroot in the cold water. Stir the dissolved arrowroot into the cooking liquid until thick and clear, about 4 minutes.

4 Remove the meat from the bone and cut it crosswise on the diagonal into thin slices. For cubes, cut crosswise into 1-inch-thick slices, then cut each slice into 1-inch strips, then 1-inch cubes. Pour the sauce over the meat and stir to coat.

5 Serve as desired. Transfer the extra portions to containers and refrigerate or freeze. Use refrigerated portions within 3 days and frozen portions within 4 months.

Turkey Chili–Stuffed Peppers with Coleslaw and Caper-Yogurt Dressing

Rachel Albert-Matesz

Prep: 20 minutes
Cooking: 2 to 5 hours

Yield: 4 (4-block) servings

Steel-cuts oats have a slightly nutty texture and rich taste that blends in with the meat so that it's almost imperceptible. They're thicker than rolled oats and lower on the glycemic index than most grains.

Block Size	Ingredients
Stuffing	
14 protein	1½ pounds ground turkey (without skin)
1 protein	1 whole egg **or** 2 egg whites
2 carbohydrate	2 tablespoons dried onion flakes
4½ carbohydrate	⅓ cup steel-cut oats **or** ¾ cup thick rolled oats
	1 tablespoon chili powder
	½ teaspoon ground chipotle (smoked dried jalapeño) **or** ground ancho **or** Anaheim pepper
	½ teaspoon finely ground sea salt
Peppers and Sauce	
2 carbohydrate	4 large green bell peppers
3 carbohydrate	3 cups chopped or crushed, no salt tomatoes with their juices (such as Eden brand)
	¼ teaspoon ground black pepper
	2 to 3 garlic cloves, minced or pressed
	½ teaspoon ground cumin

Caper-Yogurt Dressing

1 protein, 1 carbohydrate	½ cup organic, low-fat yogurt, such as Stonyfield Farms
9 fat	1 tablespoon olive oil
½ carbohydrate	1 teaspoon fructose powder
	1 teaspoon Dijon **or** honey mustard
	1 teaspoon dried dill **or** 3 tablespoons fresh minced dill
	¼ cup capers, drained

Coleslaw

1 carbohydrate	4 cups shredded cabbage
1 carbohydrate	1 cup shredded carrot
½ carbohydrate	¾ cup minced sweet white onions
½ carbohydrate	1 cup celery, finely minced
7 fat	21 walnut halves, lightly toasted and chopped

Instructions

1 In a medium bowl, combine the stuffing ingredients. Mix with clean, bare hands to evenly distribute, divide the mixture into four portions, and shape it loosely into balls.

2 Slice the tops off the peppers, removing as little flesh as possible. Remove the seeds and membrane. Poke a hole in the bottom of each pepper with a fork to allow steam to enter. Stuff the peppers with the stuffing and place them upright in a 4- to 5-quart slow cooker. In a medium bowl, combine the tomatoes, pepper, garlic, and cumin. Pour the mixture over the peppers, cover, and cook on LOW for 4 to 5 hours or HIGH for 2 to 2½ hours.

3 In a large bowl, combine the caper-yogurt dressing ingredients. Add the coleslaw ingredients and toss thoroughly. Marinate the coleslaw in the refrigerator for several hours to soften. Stir well before serving.

4 To serve, pour ¼ of the red sauce over each pepper. Serve the coleslaw on the side.

Turkey Chowder, Spring Greens, and Sun-Dried Tomatoes with Berry Salad

Rachel Albert-Matesz

Prep: 25 minutes
Cooking: 3 to 8 hours

Yield: 4 (4-block) meals

I replaced leftover Thanksgiving turkey with uncooked turkey and bacon with liquid smoke seasoning and omitted the butternut squash from a recipe in Frances Towner Giedt's *Crockery Favorites.*

Block Size	Ingredients
Berry Salad	
4 carbohydrate	One 16-ounce bag frozen Private Selection Berry Medley
	1 teaspoon pure vanilla extract
2 carbohydrate	4 teaspoons fructose powder
4 fat	12 lightly toasted walnut **or** pecan halves
Chowder	
1½ carbohydrate	16-ounce bag Freshlike Frozen Pepper Stir-Fry Mix
2 carbohydrate	½ pound baby carrots, halved
½ carbohydrate	1 cup thinly sliced celery hearts or precut sticks
16 protein	16 ounces boneless skinless turkey breast, cut into 1-inch cubes
	1 teaspoon Wright's Liquid Hickory Smoke Seasoning
	¾ teaspoon dried marjoram, crumbled
	½ teaspoon dried thyme, crumbled
	¼ teaspoon ground black pepper

	3 cups salt-free or reduced sodium chicken stock
2 carbohydrate	1 cup frozen green peas

Salad

1 carbohydrate	10 cups baby greens **or** mesclun mix, washed and spun dry
2 carbohydrate	16 oil-packed sun-dried tomato halves, drained and sliced, oil reserved

Dressing

12 fat	4 teaspoons extra-virgin olive oil (from the sun-dried tomato jar)
1 carbohydrate	1½ teaspoons honey or agavé nectar
	2½ tablespoons organic red wine vinegar
	2 teaspoons Dijon mustard

Instructions

1 The night before serving, pour the frozen fruit into a nonmetallic bowl. Drizzle with the vanilla and sprinkle with the fructose powder. Cover and thaw in refrigerator overnight. Chop the nuts and set aside.

2 Layer the chowder ingredients (except the peas) in a 3½- to 5-quart slow cooker. Do not stir. Cover and cook on LOW for 6 to 8 hours or HIGH for 3 to 4 hours.

3 Fifteen minutes before serving, add the peas to the slow cooker. If cooking on LOW, raise setting to HIGH. Cover and cook until the peas are tender and cooked through, about 15 minutes.

4 Layer the salad ingredients in a large serving bowl. In a small bowl, whisk together the dressing ingredients. Pour the dressing over the salad, toss to coat, and divide the salad among 4 serving plates.

5 Stir the thawed berries and divide them among 4 small custard cups. Garnish with the nuts. Ladle the chowder into 4 serving bowls and serve with the salad and berries.

Pork and Black Bean Stew with Broccoli-Cauliflower and Pimiento-Olive Salad

Rachel Albert-Matesz

Prep: 25 minutes   **Yield:**   4 (4-block) servings
Cooking: 3 to 8 hours

Feel free to substitute small red beans or navy beans for the black beans. If you like it hot, add hot sauce at the table.

Block Size	Ingredients
Stew	
1 carbohydrate	1½ cups onion, cut into ½-inch dice
2 carbohydrate	½ pound baby carrots, halved
½ carbohydrate	1 yellow bell pepper, halved, seeded, and diced
2 carbohydrate	One 14½-ounce can Eden no-salt-added diced whole tomatoes, with juices
16 protein	16 ounces boneless pork, trimmed of visible fat, cut into ½- to 1-inch cubes
	½ teaspoon ground cumin
	¼ to ½ teaspoon ground chipotle (smoked dried jalapeño) **or** 1 teaspoon hot sauce containing chipotle
	1 large or 2 medium garlic cloves, minced
	2 teaspoons Wright's Liquid Hickory Smoke Seasoning
8 carbohydrate	2 cups canned black beans, cooked and drained
	1 tablespoon tamari soy sauce **or** dark miso (optional)
	½ cup minced fresh cilantro **or** parsley

Vegetables

	¾ to 1 cup filtered water
1 carbohydrate	4 cups fresh raw cauliflower florets (may be precut)
1 carbohydrate	4 cups fresh raw broccoli florets (may be precut)
8 fat	2⅔ teaspoons extra-virgin olive oil
½ carbohydrate	2½ tablespoons balsamic vinegar
8 fat	24 pimento-stuffed olives, thinly sliced

Instructions

1 Combine the stew ingredients (except the tamari or miso and cilantro or parsley) in a 3½- to 4-quart slow cooker. Stir, cover, and cook on LOW 6 to 8 hours or HIGH 3 to 4 hours, or until the pork is tender.

2 To make the vegetables, in a covered 2- to 3-quart saucepan fitted with a metal steamer basket over medium heat, boil the water. Add cauliflower and broccoli, cover, and steam until tender, 5 to 8 minutes. In a small bowl, combine the olive oil, vinegar, and olives. Transfer the steamed vegetables to a medium bowl. Toss with dressing, divide among 4 small bowls.

3 Dissolve the miso or tamari into ½ cup of the stew, add the mixture back to the cooker, and stir. Ladle the stew into 4 large serving bowls and garnish with the cilantro or parsley. Serve with the vegetables.

Slow-Cooked Pork Ragout with Spinach, Olive, and Tangerine Salad

Rachel Albert-Matesz

Prep: 30 minutes   **Yield:**   4 (4-block) meals
Cooking: 3½ to 9 hours

I made minor modifications of a pork ragout recipe found in Frances Towner Giedt's *Heartland Cooking: Crockery Favorites.* Spinach, olives, and tangerines team up for an intriguing side salad.

Block Size	Ingredients
Pork Ragout	
16 protein	1 pound pork loin, trimmed of fat, cut in 1½-inch pieces
1 carbohydrate	⅓ cup fresh orange juice
½ carbohydrate	Juice of ½ lime
1 carbohydrate	1½ cups coarsely chopped red onion
	1 large garlic clove, minced or pressed
	2 ounces canned or jarred diced green chilies, drained
	½ teaspoon dried oregano, crumbled
	½ teaspoon ground cumin
	½ teaspoon hot or mild Hungarian paprika
	⅛ teaspoon ground cayenne or ancho pepper
	⅛ teaspoon ground black pepper, or to taste
Beans	
8 carbohydrate	2 cups cooked, drained, unsalted organic black beans, about 1½ (15-ounce) cans

⅓ cup chicken stock or broth, or as
   needed to moisten

1 tablespoon tamari soy sauce (optional)

½ cup minced scallions (green onions),
   parsley, or cilantro

Spinach Salad

1 carbohydrate	10 cups baby spinach or spring greens, washed and spun dry
4 carbohydrate	4 small tangerines **or** clementines, peeled and sectioned
7 fat	21 pitted black olives, thinly sliced
9 fat	1 tablespoon extra-virgin olive oil
½ carbohydrate	Juice of ½ lime
	2 teaspoons Dijon mustard
	½ teaspoon lemon pepper

Instructions

1 Combine the pork ragout ingredients in 3½- to 5-quart slow cooker. Stir, cover, and cook on LOW for 7 to 9 hours or HIGH for 3½ to 4½ hours. If cooking on HIGH, stir once during the final hour of cooking.

2 About 15 minutes before serving, warm the beans in a saucepan or heatproof bowl in a toaster oven with enough broth to moisten. Add the tamari if desired. Stir occasionally.

3 Wash the baby spinach or greens and spin dry. Divide among 4 serving plates. Top with the tangerine or clementine slices. Sprinkle with the olives. In a small bowl, whisk together the olive oil, lime juice, mustard, and lemon pepper and drizzle the dressing over the salad.

4 Ladle the ragout into one side of each of 4 shallow serving bowls. Spoon the beans into the other side of each bowl. Garnish with chopped scallions (green onions), parsley, or cilantro and serve.

Moroccan Lamb and Lentil Stew with Cauliflower, Pepper, and Olive Salad

Rachel Albert-Matesz

Prep: 20 minutes   **Yield:**   4 (4-block) servings
Cooking: 3 to 8 hours

This stew is a takeoff on a soup from Lou Seibert Pappas' *Extra-Special Crockery Pot Recipes.* Out of lentils? Substitute small white (navy) beans or chickpeas. Instead of lamb, try pork.

Block Size	Ingredients
Stew	
16 protein	16 ounces boneless lamb meat, trimmed of fat and cubed
	½ teaspoon ground cumin
	1 teaspoon finely ground ginger **or** ¼ teaspoon dried ginger
	⅛ to ¼ teaspoon ground cayenne **or** ancho pepper
	1 large garlic clove, minced
	2 bay leaves
2 carbohydrate	½ pound baby carrots, halved
1 carbohydrate	1½ cups red onion, cut into ½-inch dice
½ carbohydrate	½ cup chopped celery
8 carbohydrate	2 cups drained, canned, cooked unsalted lentils
2 carbohydrate	One 14½-ounce can Eden no-salt-added, diced whole tomatoes, with juices
	1 tablespoon dark miso **or** tamari soy sauce (optional)
	½ cup minced fresh cilantro

Vegetables

	¾ cup filtered water
1½ carbohydrate	One 16-ounce bag frozen cauliflower **or** 4 cups fresh, raw cauliflower florets
1 carbohydrate	½ of a 16-ounce bag Freshlike Frozen Pepper Stir-Fry (green, red, and yellow bell pepper strips with onions) **or** 2 fresh yellow bell peppers, halved, seeded, and diced
6 fat	2 teaspoons extra-virgin olive oil
	2 teaspoons organic red wine vinegar
	½ teaspoon lemon pepper
10 fat	30 pitted black olives, thinly sliced

Instructions

1 Combine the stew ingredients (except the miso or tamari and cilantro) in a 3½- to 4-quart slow cooker. Stir, cover, and cook on LOW for 6 to 8 hours or HIGH for 3 to 4 hours, or until the lamb is tender. Remove and discard the bay leaves.

2 To make the vegetables, in a covered 2- to 3-quart saucepan fitted with a metal steamer basket over medium heat, bring the water to a boil. Add the cauliflower and peppers to the steamer, cover, and steam until tender, 5 to 8 minutes. In a small bowl, whisk together the olive oil, vinegar, and pepper.

3 Dissolve the miso or tamari into ½ cup of stew, add the mixture back to cooker, and stir. Ladle the stew into 4 large serving bowls and garnish with the cilantro. Transfer the steamed vegetables to a medium bowl and toss with the dressing and olives. Divide among 4 shallow small bowls and serve.

Three-Bean Beef Chili with Green Salad and Guacamole

Rachel Albert-Matesz

Prep: 20 minutes
Cooking: 7 to 9 hours

Yield: 4 (4-block) servings

This stew is a takeoff on one found in *Smart Crockery Cooking* by Carol Munsen. You can start it in a slow cooker just before you leave for work in the morning, or you can take cooked chili to work in a thermos bottle.

Block Size	Ingredients
1 carbohydrate	1½ cups diced fresh **or** thawed frozen onion
3 carbohydrate	¾ cup no-salt added, drained, canned kidney beans
3 carbohydrate	¾ cup no-salt added, drained, canned black beans
3 carbohydrate	¾ cup no-salt added, drained, canned pinto black beans
12 protein	18 ounces lean ground beef
1 carbohydrate	2 cups diced fresh **or** thawed frozen bell pepper strips
	3 garlic cloves, minced
	1 tablespoon chili powder blend
	½ teaspoon ground cumin
	⅛ teaspoon ground allspice
	⅛ teaspoon ground coriander
	½ tablespoon red wine vinegar
2 carbohydrate	2 cups diced no-salt plum tomatoes, with juices
	¼ cup chopped fresh cilantro

Salad

½ carbohydrate	5 cups romaine lettuce
½ carbohydrate	2 cups thinly sliced red radish
1 carbohydrate	2 cups thinly sliced celery hearts
4 protein	4 ounces shredded low-fat cheese (1 cup)

Guacamole

16 fat	1 cup guacamole **or** mashed avocado
1 carbohydrate	⅓ cup lemon **or** lime juice
	Hot sauce, to taste

Instructions

1 Layer the chili ingredients (except the cilantro) in a 3½-quart slow cooker. Cover and cook on LOW for 7 to 9 hours.

2 Divide the salad vegetables among 4 large dinner plates. Top with the cheese. In a small bowl, mash the guacamole or avocado with the lemon or lime juice and hot sauce. Place a dollop of the guacamole on top of each salad.

3 Divide the chili among 4 large soup bowls, garnish with cilantro, and serve immediately.

Variations

Replace beef with buffalo (bison) or ground turkey.

Beef and Barley Stew with Greek Salad

Rachel Albert-Matesz

Prep: 25 minutes   **Yield:**   4 (4-block) servings
Cooking: 9 to 11 hours

Start this stew, an adaptation of one by Mable Hoffman, before leaving for work in the morning. Toss the salad just before serving. Pack the leftovers for lunch the next day or save them for supper.

Block Size	Ingredients
Stew	
12 protein	¾ pound beef stew meat or round steak, cubed
8 carbohydrate	¼ cup pearl barley, rinsed and drained
1 carbohydrate	1½ cups diced onion
1 carbohydrate	1 small turnip, peeled, cut into ½-inch cubes (1½ cups)
2 carbohydrate	2 cups diced carrots or halved baby carrots
½ carbohydrate	1 cup thinly sliced celery ribs with leaves
	One 14-ounce can low-salt beef broth **or** homemade stock
	1 teaspoon dried thyme leaves, crumbled
	½ teaspoon dried sage
	½ teaspoon ground cumin
	¼ teaspoon ground black pepper
	2 garlic cloves, minced or crushed
	1 bay leaf
	1 tablespoon tamari soy sauce **or** dark miso paste

Salad

¾ carbohydrate	7½ cups romaine washed, spun dry
½ carbohydrate	¾ cup red onion or Walla Walla Sweet **or** Vidalia onion, cut into thin rings or half-moons
1 carbohydrate	2 cored tomatoes, diced
¼ carbohydrate	½ cup thinly sliced yellow bell pepper
7 fat	21 pitted black olives, thinly sliced
4 protein	4 ounces reduced-fat feta cheese, crumbled

Dressing

9 fat	1 tablespoon extra-virgin olive oil
½ carbohydrate	2½ tablespoons balsamic vinegar
½ carbohydrate	2½ tablespoons lemon juice
	2 tablespoons chicken stock **or** broth
	¼ teaspoon ground black pepper
	1 teaspoon anchovy paste

Instructions

1 Layer the stew ingredients (except the tamari or miso) in 3½- to 4-quart slow cooker. Cover and cook on LOW for 9 to 11 hours, until the beef and barley are tender.

2 Just before serving, layer the salad ingredients on 4 large dinner plates.

3 Combine the dressing ingredients in a small jar. Cover and shake, then pour over the salad.

4 Dissolve the tamari or miso in ½ cup of stew. Add the mixture back to the cooker and stir. Spoon the stew into 4 large soup bowls and serve.

Beef and Walnut Ratatouille with Red Wine and Feta and Broccoli, Cauliflower, and Capers

Rachel Albert-Matesz

Prep: 20 minutes
Cooking: 3 to 8 hours

Yield: 4 (4-block) meals

Ratatouille is a classic eggplant, tomato, and zucchini stew made with garlic and Italian herbs. The addition of ground beef turns it into a main dish and red wine adds a more robust flavor.

Block Size	Ingredients
Ratatouille	
12 protein	18 ounces lean ground beef
7 fat	21 walnut halves, lightly toasted and chopped
1 protein	1 whole egg **or** 2 egg whites
	¼ teaspoon ground black **or** red pepper
2 carbohydrate	1 cup red wine
2 carbohydrate	3 cups red **or** white onions, cut into thin half-moons
2 carbohydrate	2 cups cubed **or** diced fresh or canned no-salt-added tomatoes, with juices
2 carbohydrate	4 cups zucchini, trimmed and cut into 2-inch cubes
½ carbohydrate	1 yellow bell pepper, halved, seeded, cut into 1-inch dice
3 carbohydrate	4½ cups eggplant, peeled, cut into 1½-inch cubes
	1 bay leaf
	3 garlic cloves, minced **or** pressed

	½ teaspoon dried, crumbled thyme **or**
	3 sprigs fresh thyme
	1 teaspoon dried basil
1 carbohydrate	2 teaspoons fructose powder
	Freshly ground black pepper, to taste
	¼ cup minced fresh parsley **or** basil leaves
3 protein	3 ounces reduced-fat feta cheese, crumbled

Broccoli and Cauliflower

1½ carbohydrate	One 16-ounce package frozen broccoli
1½ carbohydrate	One 16-ounce package frozen cauliflower
9 fat	1 tablespoon extra-virgin olive oil
	¼ cup capers, drained and minced
	1 teaspoon dried dill
½ carbohydrate	Juice of ½ lemon

Instructions

1 In a small bowl, mix the ground beef, walnuts, egg, and pepper. Form into table-spoon-size balls.

2 Add the wine, onions, tomatoes, zucchini, bell pepper, eggplant, bay leaf, garlic, thyme, basil, and fructose to a 3½- to 5-quart slow cooker and stir. Arrange the meatballs on top of the vegetables. Cover and cook on LOW for 6 to 8 hours or HIGH for 3 to 4 hours.

3 About 15 minutes before serving, add 2 cups water to a 3-quart saucepan. Insert a collapsible metal steamer. Cover, bring to boil over medium heat, and add the broccoli and cauliflower. Cover and steam until the vegetables are easily pierced with a fork, 5 to 7 minutes. In a large bowl, whisk the olive oil, capers, dill, and lemon juice. Drain the vegetables and add them to the dressing. Toss to coat and divide among 4 serving bowls.

4 Before serving the stew, discard the bay leaf. Add pepper, stir, and taste. Ladle into 4 large soup bowls. Garnish with the parsley or basil and feta and serve with the vegetables.

Beef Goulash with Cabbage, Avocado "Sour Cream," and Apple-Berry Sauce

Rachel Albert-Matesz

Prep: 20 to 30 minutes   **Yield:**   4 (4-block) meals
Cooking: 4 to 10 hours

This is a Zoned rendition of a recipe from *New Flavors from Your Crockery Cooker,* put out by *Better Homes & Gardens.*

Block Size	Ingredients
Goulash	
4 carbohydrate	1⅓ cups potato, cut into 1-inch cubes
2 carbohydrate	3 cups onion, diced or cut into half-moon slices
	2 garlic cloves, minced
	1 bay leaf
16 protein	1 pound stew beef **or** top eye **or** sirloin tip steak, cubed
	1 cup no-salt added beef stock **or** broth
2 carbohydrate	2 cups diced, canned, no-salt tomatoes **or** chunky tomatoes with garlic and green chili peppers, with juices
1 carbohydrate	¼ cup no-salt-added tomato paste
	2 tablespoons Hungarian paprika (mild or hot)
	1 teaspoon caraway **or** fennel seed
	¼ teaspoon ground black pepper
	½ teaspoon sea salt
Cabbage	
	½ to 1 cup filtered water
2 carbohydrate	8 cups shredded red and/or green cabbage

Avocado "Sour Cream"

12 fat	¾ cup seeded, diced avocado
1 carbohydrate	Juice of 1 lime

Apple-Berry Sauce

4 carbohydrate	2 cups Santa Cruz Naturals blackberry applesauce
4 fat	12 lightly toasted walnuts, coarsely chopped

Instructions

1 Layer the potato, onion, garlic, bay leaf, and beef in a 3½- to 5-quart slow cooker. In a medium bowl, combine the broth, tomatoes and juice, tomato paste, paprika, caraway or fennel seed, pepper, and salt. Stir and add to the slow cooker. Cover and cook on LOW for 8 to 10 hours or HIGH for 4 to 5 hours.

2 Bring the water to boil over medium heat in a 2-quart saucepan fitted with a metal vegetable steamer/basket. Add the cabbage to the steamer. Cover and steam until tender, 5 to 7 minutes.

3 Whip the avocado and lime in a food processor or with an electric mixer until smooth.

4 Divide the applesauce among 4 small dishes and garnish with the nuts. Divide the cabbage among 4 large soup bowls, top with the goulash and the avocado "sour cream," and serve.

Variation

Replace cabbage with broccoli and/or cauliflower florets.

Beef 'n' Oat–Stuffed Peppers with Cauliflower, Artichoke Hearts, and Walnuts

Rachel Albert-Matesz

Prep: 20 minutes
Cooking: 2 to 5 hours

Yield: 4 (4-block) servings

Steel-cut oats are the surprise ingredient in this Zone-friendly version of an American classic. They have more texture, body, and flavor, than rolled oats.

Block Size	Ingredients
Stuffing	
15 protein	22 ounces lean ground beef **or** bison
1 protein	1 whole egg **or** 2 egg whites
2 carbohydrate	2 tablespoons dried onion flakes
6 carbohydrate	½ cup steel-cut oats **or** 1 cup thick rolled oats
	¼ cup minced fresh **or** 1 tablespoon dried parsley
	1 teaspoon dried basil, crumbled
	¾ teaspoon dried oregano, crumbled
	¼ teaspoon ground red pepper, or to taste
	½ teaspoon finely ground sea salt **or** 1 tablespoon tamari soy sauce
Peppers and Sauce	
2 carbohydrate	4 extra-large green bell peppers
3 carbohydrate	3 cups chopped **or** crushed, no-salt tomatoes with juices (such as Eden brand)
	¼ teaspoon ground black pepper
	½ teaspoon ground cumin
	2 to 3 garlic cloves, minced or pressed

Cauliflower and Artichoke Hearts

2 carbohydrate	Two 16-ounce bags thawed frozen cauliflower
1 carbohydrate	One 14-ounce bag Private Selection frozen artichoke hearts
	2 teaspoons Dijon mustard
	¼ teaspoon ground black pepper
	2 tablespoons red wine vinegar
	1 tablespoon tamari soy sauce **or** ume plum vinegar
9 fat	1 tablespoon extra-virgin olive oil
7 fat	21 walnut halves, lightly toasted, then chopped

Instructions

1 In a medium bowl, combine the stuffing ingredients. Mix with clean bare hands to evenly distribute, divide into four portions, and shape loosely into balls.

2 Slice the tops off the peppers, removing as little flesh as possible. Remove the seeds and membrane. Poke a hole in the bottom of each pepper with a fork to allow the steam to enter. Stuff the peppers with the filling and place upright in a 4- to 5-quart slow cooker. In a medium bowl, mix the tomatoes, pepper, cumin, and garlic. Pour the mixture over the peppers. Cover and cook on LOW for 4 to 5 hours or HIGH for 2 to 2 ½ hours.

3 About 10 minutes before serving, insert a collapsible metal steamer into a 3-quart saucepan containing 2 cups of water. Cover and bring to boil over medium heat. Add the frozen vegetables to the steamer, cover, and steam until easily pierced with a fork, 5 to 7 minutes. Combine the remaining ingredients in a large serving bowl. Drain the vegetables, add them to a bowl with the olive oil, and toss to coat. Divide among 4 dinner plates. Garnish with the nuts.

4 Place a stuffed pepper and a portion of the tomato sauce on each dinner plate and serve.

Note: Transfer the frozen meat to a pan in the refrigerator 24 to 36 hours before you need it so that it has ample time to thaw.

Beef-Mushroom Stew with Spinach-Orange Salad and Raspberry Vinaigrette

Rachel Albert-Matesz

Prep: 20 minutes   **Yield:**   4 (4-block) meals
Cooking: 3 to 8 hours

This recipe is a variation on one found on the website for Laura's Lean Beef (www.lauraslean-beef.com). I changed the proportion of ingredients to make them Zone favorable. The sweet salad makes a tasty first or second course.

Block Size	Ingredients
Beef and Mushroom Stew	
16 protein	1 pound stew meat **or** top eye **or** sirloin tip steak, cut into 2-inch cubes
2 carbohydrate	3 cups diced onion
½ carbohydrate	2 cups thinly sliced button, cremini, or shiitake mushrooms, stems removed
4 carbohydrate	8 ounces raw potato, cut into 2-inch cubes
½ carbohydrate	4 celery stalks, cut into 1-inch pieces
	1 large bay leaf
	2 large garlic cloves, coarsely chopped
	1 tablespoon tamari soy sauce (optional)
	1 teaspoon Wright's Natural Liquid Hickory Smoke Seasoning
	1 teaspoon dried thyme, crumbled
	½ teaspoon ground black pepper
	½ teaspoon ground cumin
1 carbohydrate	½ cup dry red wine
	3 cups no-salt-added beef stock **or** broth
1½ carbohydrate	2 tablespoons arrowroot **or** cornstarch
	¼ cup cold water **or** beef stock

Spinach-Orange Salad

½ carbohydrate	10 cups baby spinach, washed and spun dry
4 carbohydrate	2 seedless oranges, peeled, seeded, sectioned, and halved
12 fat	36 hazelnuts **or** pecans, lightly toasted and coarsely chopped
2 carbohydrate, 4 fat	½ cup Annie's Naturals Raspberry Vinaigrette Dressing

Instructions

1 In the order listed, layer the stew ingredients (except the arrowroot or cornstarch and water or stock) in a 3½- to 4-quart slow cooker. Cover and cook on LOW for 6 to 8 hours or HIGH for 3 to 4 hours. Discard the bay leaf.

2 In a small bowl, dissolve the arrowroot or cornstarch in the ¼ cup water or stock. Transfer most of the liquid from the cooker to a medium saucepan over medium heat. Add the arrowroot mixture. Simmer, stirring constantly, until the sauce is thickened to the desired consistency. Pour the sauce back into the stew, stir, and adjust the seasonings. Ladle the stew into 4 serving bowls.

3 Layer the spinach, oranges, and nuts in a large bowl. Toss with the vinaigrette, divide among 4 large salad plates or bowls, and serve with the stew.

Minestrone Stew with Pear, Raspberry, Walnut, and Feta Salad

Rachel Albert-Matesz

Prep: 25 minutes   **Yield:**   4 (4-block) servings
Cooking: 7 to 8 hours

I omitted macaroni from this minestrone to keep the carbohydrates in check. Pears and berries add a sweet taste and cool contrast to salad greens. Walnuts add crunch, while the feta adds a salty and tangy contrast. You can use mesclun greens or some other salad mix.

Block Size	Ingredients
Stew	
12 protein	¾ pound beef chuck steak, cut into ½-inch cubes
1 carbohydrate	1½ cups diced onion
1 carbohydrate	1 cup diced carrots
4 carbohydrate	1 cup cooked, drained unsalted chickpeas
	One 14-ounce can low salt beef broth **or** homemade stock
½ carbohydrate	2 cups shredded green cabbage
¼ carbohydrate	½ cup thinly sliced celery
	1 tablespoon chopped fresh **or** 1 teaspoon dried basil
	1 tablespoon chopped fresh **or** 1 teaspoon dried parsley
	¼ teaspoon ground black pepper
	2 garlic cloves, minced or crushed
	1 bay leaf
	½ teaspoon sea salt (optional)
2 carbohydrate	One 14½-ounce can Eden no-salt-added diced whole tomatoes, with juices

Salad

¾ carbohydrate	7½ cups baby greens **or** mesclun mix, washed and spun dry
2 carbohydrate	2 cup fresh raspberries, washed and spun dry
4 carbohydrate	2 small pears, washed, halved, cored, and thinly sliced
6 fat	18 walnut halves, lightly toasted and coarsely chopped
4 protein	4 ounces feta cheese, crumbled
10 fat	⅓ cup Nayonnaise (soy-based sandwich spread)
	1 tablespoon poppy seeds
¼ carbohydrate	1½ tablespoons lemon juice
¼ carbohydrate	1½ tablespoons orange juice

Instructions

1 Layer the stew ingredients in a 3½- to 4-quart slow cooker. Cover and cook on LOW for 7 to 8 hours, until beef is tender.

2 Just before serving, layer the greens, raspberries, pears, walnuts, and feta on 4 large plates.

3 In a small bowl, blend the Nayonnaise, poppy seeds, lemon juice, and orange juice. Pour the dressing over the salad, ladle the stew into 4 large soup bowls, and serve.

Variation

Use half chickpeas and half kidney beans.

Timber Creek Buffalo and Black Bean Chili with Jicama and Guacamole

Rachel Albert-Matesz

Prep: 25 minutes   **Yield:**   4 (4-block) servings
Cooking: 3 to 7 hours

Timber Creek Farms of Yorkville, Illinois, a company that delivers organic foods to consumers by truck and mail-order, provided the inspiration for this chili. Feel free to replace buffalo with beefalo or lean ground beef, or use Muir Glen fire-roasted tomatoes.

Block Size	Ingredients
Chili	
1 carbohydrate	1½ cups finely diced onion
1 carbohydrate	1 cup diced carrots **or** ¼ pound halved baby carrots
½ carbohydrate	1 green bell pepper, seeded and diced
½ carbohydrate	1 yellow or red bell pepper, seeded and diced
5 carbohydrate	One 15-ounce can Eden no-salt-added black beans, drained
16 protein	16 ounces buffalo stew meat **or** ground meat, thawed
	2 garlic cloves, minced or crushed
	1 teaspoon chili powder (mild or hot)
	1 teaspoon ground coriander
	1 teaspoon dried basil, crumbled
	¼ teaspoon ground chipotle, ancho, or Anaheim pepper
2 carbohydrate	One 14½-ounce can Eden no-salt-added diced whole tomatoes, with juices
	1 tablespoon tamari soy sauce **or** dark miso

| 1 carbohydrate | 10 cups romaine **or** mixed salad greens |
| | ¼ cup chopped fresh cilantro **or** parsley for garnish |

Jicama

| 1 carbohydrate | 2½ cups jicama, peeled and cut into finger-long sticks |
| ½ carbohydrate | 2½ tablespoons lime juice |

Guacamole

16 fat	1 cup mashed avocado
½ carbohydrate	2½ tablespoons lime juice
	½ teaspoon ground cumin
	Hot sauce, to taste

Fruit

| 3 carbohydrate | 2¼ cups seedless watermelon, cubed |

Instructions

1 Layer the onion, carrots, bell peppers, beans, and buffalo in a 3½- to 4-quart slow cooker. Add the garlic, chili powder, coriander, basil, chipotle, and tomatoes. Cover and cook on LOW for 6 to 7 hours or HIGH for 3 to 3½ hours, or until the onions are tender and the meat is cooked through.

2 To make the jicama, toss it with the lime juice in a medium bowl. To make the guacamole, in a small bowl, mash the avocado, lime juice, cumin, and hot sauce.

3 Add the tamari to the chili or dissolve the miso into ½ cup of the chili, add the mixture to the cooker, and stir. Divide the lettuce among 4 large soup bowls. Spoon the chili over the lettuce and top with the cilantro or parsley. Serve the jicama and guacamole on the side. Serve the watermelon for dessert.

Zoned Beef and Vegetable Stew with Spring Green and Strawberry Salad

Rachel Albert-Matesz

Prep: 20 minutes   **Yield:**   4 (4-block) meals
Cooking: 3 to 8 hours

This recipe is based on one found on the website for Laura's Lean Beef (www.lauraslean-beef.com). The proportion of ingredients have been changed to make them Zone favorable. The sweet salad makes a tasty first or second course.

Block Size	Ingredients
Stew	
16 protein	1 pound stew meat **or** top eye **or** sirloin tip steak, cut into 2-inch cubes
1 carbohydrate	1½ cups diced onion
2 carbohydrate	2 cups diced, canned, no-salt tomatoes, with juices
4 carbohydrate	1-pound bag baby carrots
3 carbohydrate	1 cup sliced water chestnuts
½ carbohydrate	1 sweet yellow **or** red bell pepper, diced **or** 1 cup frozen bell pepper strips, thawed
½ carbohydrate	1 cup thinly sliced celery
	1 tablespoon tamari soy sauce **or** ½ teaspoon sea salt
	2 garlic cloves, minced **or** ½ teaspoon garlic powder
	1 bay leaf
	1 tablespoon dried basil **or** Italian herb blend
	2 cups no-salt-added beef stock
	1½ tablespoons chopped fresh parsley

Salad

1 carbohydrate	10 cups baby greens **or** mesclun mix, washed and spun dry
2 carbohydrate	2 cups fresh strawberries, hulled and thinly sliced
12 fat	36 pecan halves, lightly toasted and coarsely crumbled
2 carbohydrate, 4 fat	½ cup Annie's Naturals Raspberry Vinaigrette Dressing

Instructions

1 In the order listed, layer the stew ingredients (except the parsley) in a 3½- to 4-quart slow cooker. Cover and cook on LOW for 6 to 8 hours or HIGH for 3 to 4 hours. Discard the bay leaf before serving.

2 Just before serving, layer the greens, strawberries, and pecans on 4 large salad plates or in bowls. Top with the dressing.

3 Ladle the stew into wide, shallow soup bowls. Garnish with the parsley and serve.

Variations

Replace beef with lean, trimmed pork.

Vegetarian Kidney Bean and Walnut Chili with Salad Greens and Corn

Rachel Albert-Matesz

Prep: 25 minutes   **Yield:**   4 (4-block) servings
Cooking: 5 to 6 hours

Start this stew in a slow cooker just before you run errands, so it's ready for supper when you arrive home, or simmer it on top of the stove while you toss a salad in the evening.

Block Size	Ingredients
Chili	
2 carbohydrate	3 cups onions, cut in half-moons
8 carbohydrate	2 cups no-salt-added, cooked, drained canned kidney beans
6 fat	18 walnut halves, coarsely chopped
	3 garlic cloves, minced
	1 bay leaf
	1½ tablespoons chili powder
	1 teaspoon ground cumin
	¼ teaspoon ground chipotle (smoked dried jalapeño) **or** hot sauce
2 carbohydrate	2 cups chopped, canned no-salt-added tomatoes with juices **or** one 14½-ounce can Eden diced whole tomatoes
12 protein	12 soy hot dogs, thinly sliced
	1 to 2 tablespoons tamari soy sauce **or** dark miso

Salad

1 carbohydrate	10 cups spring salad mix **or** baby greens mix
10 fat	⅔ cup mashed avocado **or** guacamole
4 protein	4 ounces low-fat cheddar or jack cheese, shredded (1 cup)

Corn

3 carbohydrate	1 ear sweet corn, cut into 4 pieces
	⅓ cup filtered water

Instructions

1 Layer the onions, beans, walnuts, garlic, bay leaf, chili powder, cumin, chipotle, and tomatoes in a 3½- to 4-quart slow cooker. Cover and cook on LOW for 5 to 6 hours. Add the soy hot dog slices 1 hour before serving. Just before serving, dissolve the tamari or miso into ½ cup of chili, add it back to the cooker, and stir.

2 Divide the salad greens among 4 large dinner plates. Top with the avocado or guacamole and cheese.

3 Place the sweet corn and water in a small saucepan. Cover and bring to boil over medium-high heat. Lower the heat to medium and steam for 5 to 8 minutes, or until tender. Transfer to serving plates. Divide the chili among 4 soup bowls and serve with the salads.

Variations

Replace kidney beans with cooked lentils.

10

Special Occasions
in the Zone

If life were made up of simple breakfasts, lunches, dinners, and snacks, we feel confident that, having read this far, you could live your life comfortably in the Zone. But life is made up of so much more. Take the family barbecue, traditionally featuring mounds of potato salad, hamburger buns, corn on the cob, and beer—a virtual Zone land mine. And what do you serve at a dinner party? Or how can you make sure you stay in the Zone when invited to a dinner party? Dining out gives one pause, too. Portions are usually way too big, with mounds of pasta or rice or potatoes or bread. Other Zone roadblocks traditionally occur between Thanksgiving and Christmas, a time that usually turns into an overeating marathon. Finally, what do you do when your buddies ask you to go out drinking? I'll bet you think those good times are over now that you are in the Zone—but that's not the case at all.

THE BARBECUE

There's nothing potentially more Zoneful than a barbecue. We often hold summer barbecues on our patio, bringing together family members and friends. If our older daughter Kelly is home for a visit, everyone is really in for a culinary treat; she's a terrific cook. At a recent barbecue, she marinated chicken, shark, mahi-mahi, and swordfish. We also had an emu steak and some aged free-range beef.

One of Kelly's marinades was simply delicious.

Kelly's Marinade

2 tablespoons chopped cilantro

2 cloves garlic, minced

1 tablespoon fish sauce

2 teaspoons soy sauce

Juice of 1 lime

Marinate meats or fish for 30 minutes in the refrigerator.

She also likes Baja Lime/Tamatillo Marinade from Trader Joe's.

We ate vegetables wrapped in foil and seasoned with ginger, soy sauce, and lime. If you leave space in the foil packet, the steam makes the veggies very tender. Both fresh and frozen vegetables work well. You can find recipes on the Reynold's Wrap package for both the grill and the oven, or go to www.reynoldskitchens.com for more recipes.

I often turn to product websites to learn creative ways to cook with lentils, barley, and steel-cut oatmeal. At the site www.Mccanns.ie I found a recipe for Irish Oatmeal Risotto that proved to be a hit at our barbecue. I simplified the recipe significantly. The recipe yields about 10 blocks of carbohydrate and about 2 blocks of protein. Just make sure you add enough protein to balance it out.

Irish Oatmeal Risotto

4 cups chicken or beef broth

¼ cup minced shallots

2 garlic cloves, peeled and minced, or to taste

1 cup McCann's Irish steel-cut oatmeal

1 tablespoon minced fresh parsley

1 tablespoon lemon juice

½ cup grated Parmesan cheese

Salt and pepper to taste

In a heavy saucepan, bring the broth, shallots, and garlic to a boil over medium high heat. Pour in the oats and turn heat down to low. Cover but leave the lid slightly askew to prevent boil-overs. Cook, stirring occasionally, for 30 minutes or until the oatmeal is the consistency that you like it. Remove from the heat. Stir in parsley, lemon juice, cheese, salt, and pepper. Serve hot.

—*Lynn Sears*

We served dips, but instead of chips, we supplied red and green pepper sticks and zucchini sticks. We offered fruit for dessert: mixed blueberries and raspberries, with a bowl of freshly whipped cream on the side.

Wine and beer can also be found on the Zone menu. See Alcohol in the Zone on page 356.

DINNER PARTIES

If you give a dinner party, you'll be able to choose the foods that will keep you and your guests in the Zone. When we give a dinner party, the menu almost always includes Zoned Lasagna. Our guests can't believe it's possible—but it is, and it's delicious.

Zoned Lasagna

This recipe yields 12 blocks. A typical woman would eat roughly a fourth of the lasagna; a typical man about a third. Better still, eat less than the full block requirements and add something else to the menu. But don't sweat it, just enjoy.

Block Size	Ingredients
12 fat	4 teaspoons olive oil
4 protein	2 cups frozen Morningstar Farms Veggie Recipe Crumbles
4 carbohydrate	2 cups tomato sauce
	Parsley, basil, and garlic to taste or spices of your choice
3 protein	½ cup skim ricotta cheese
1 protein	1 egg
	2 tablespoons minced parsley
	2 tablespoons Parmesan cheese
8 carbohydrate	6 no-bake lasagna noodles
4 protein	4 ounces skim mozzarella cheese, sliced

Instructions

1 Preheat the oven to 375° F.

2 In a large sauté pan over medium-high heat, heat the olive oil. Add the veggie crumbles and cook, stirring often, until hot. Add the tomato sauce and spices of your choice. Cook over medium heat until flavors blend, about 20 minutes, stirring often.

3 In a small bowl, mix the ricotta cheese, egg, parsley, and Parmesan.

4 In an 11 × 7-inch casserole dish, place a thin layer of the sauce mixture. Put 3 lasagna noodles on top, followed by half the remaining sauce mixture, half the mozzarella, and half the ricotta cheese mixture.

5 Layer on the remaining 3 lasagna noodles and the rest of the sauce mixture, mozzarella, and ricotta cheese mixture.

6 Cover the pan with foil and bake for 35 minutes, or until lasagna is bubbly and cooked through.

7 Let the lasagna rest for 15 minutes before cutting.

Variation

You may substitute 6 ounces of ground turkey for the veggie crumbles.

Another way to save time when planning a dinner party is to go to a store that specializes in prepared food. You can place your order ahead of time and pick it up the day of the party. We usually plan on broiling, barbecuing, or baking the protein part of the meal and then pick up side dishes to go along with it. Professionally created vegetable and fruit dishes can taste much better than big bowls of pasta salad or mashed potatoes.

Included in this book are several 16-block recipes that are perfect for dinner parties, including two delicious recipes for slow cooking a turkey breast. And check out the recipes for dressings and dips.

The Can-Do Zone recipes in chapter 8 consist of 8 blocks, just about right for a dinner for two, but they can be doubled or tripled to accommodate a dinner party with old classics, such as Peking Shrimp and Beef Bourguignonne that have been brought into the Zone.

HOLIDAY MEALS AND BUFFETS

Thanksgiving usually signals the beginning of a five- or six-week eating extravaganza, which ends in remorse, a seven- or eight-pound weight gain, and diet resolutions on New Year's Day. It doesn't have to be that way.

First of all, the centerpiece of Thanksgiving is the perfectly Zone-favorable turkey. Just make sure to stick to the white meat, and don't eat the skin. Vegetables can be dressed up with sauces to be a real treat. Make the traditional green bean casserole topped 1 can of condensed mushroom soup, ½ cup milk, 1 teaspoon soy sauce, and low-fat shredded cheese. Just substitute almonds for the fried onions.

Instead of making scalloped potatoes, make scalloped vegetables. Slice zucchini thin, add olive oil, milk, and cheese, and bake until the zucchini is tender. Try cold poached asparagus in a vinaigrette dressing. Make mashed cauliflower instead of mashed potatoes. Cooking it in chicken broth makes it taste great.

Remember, alcohol is treated like a carbohydrate, which means you have to have one block of protein for every drink you have. For some, that may mean a lot of turkey.

As far as the traditional stuffing, yams, and mashed potatoes—

forget about it. You'll be glad you did when you finish your dinner and are satisfied but not stuffed. We've been experimenting with some barley stuffing recipes. The first couple came out tasting like chicken-flavored gravel, but we finally found an acceptable recipe that we adapted from the website www.washingtonbarley.org.

Barley Stuffing

Block Size	Ingredients
6 fat	2 teaspoons olive oil
	½ cup sliced fresh mushrooms
	2 garlic cloves, minced
	2 tablespoons minced scallions (green onions)
	¼ teaspoon crumbled dried rosemary
	Poultry seasoning to taste
	3 cups chicken, beef, or vegetable broth
9 carbohydrate	1 cup uncooked Goya pearl barley

Instructions

In a large sauté pan over medium-high heat, heat the olive oil. Sauté the mushrooms and garlic until the mushrooms are tender, about 5 minutes. Add the scallions, rosemary, poultry seasoning, broth, and barley and bring to a boil. Cover, reduce the heat to low, and cook, stirring occasionally, 45 minutes, or until the barley is tender and the liquid is absorbed.

Note: You'll have to add 3 fat blocks and be sure to balance with protein (i.e. turkey).

You can use that recipe as a base and add your favorite stuffing ingredients, except bread, of course. Try experimenting for some week-night meal prior to Thanksgiving so that you can make adjustments.

What about the pumpkin pie? I'm going to tell you a secret. Barry always ends his perfectly zoned Thanksgiving dinner with a small piece of pumpkin pie . . . and a big slice of skinless turkey breast. It kind of grosses people out to see the pie and turkey on the same plate, but it works for him. As he always says, "If you're going to talk the talk, you have to walk the walk."

—*Lynn Sears*

If you're planning a holiday party, a buffet is an ideal way to stay in the Zone. Serve shrimp, sliced deli meats, skinless chicken or turkey breast, baked ham, and cheeses. Veggies and good-tasting dips are also fun and healthful. Again, if you think you might be going to a home in which nothing Zoneful will be served, offer to bring some veggies and a dip and some cheese.

In any case, have a Zone-favorable snack before you leave for the party. We always have a Zone snack before we go to someone else's house for a holiday dinner or party because it dulls the appetite, and we're not as tempted to overindulge in the Zone-unfavorable goodies. It's also a good idea to have a Zone snack before you go food shopping. Grab a piece of string cheese and a handful of grapes before you leave.

RESTAURANTS

You can dine out just about anywhere and be in the Zone. Just follow these simple guidelines.

- Pass on the rolls and ask for a side salad. It takes quite a lot of lettuce to add up to one block, which means you only have to count the fat in the dressing. Enjoy the salad and have a glass of wine (one block of carbohydrate), while your unenlightened friends chomp down on the rolls. Feel pity for them. When the server asks you if you want potatoes, rice, or pasta, say "none of the above." Ask for extra vegetables instead. We have found that most servers are happy to oblige. Even with double vegetables, you'll probably have another block to spare. You can either have another glass of wine or buy a dessert for the entire table and have a tiny piece. Also, make sure you eat a portion of protein the size and the depth of the palm of your hand. In most restaurants you will be served far too much protein. Ask for the rest to be wrapped up and enjoy it the next day for lunch. That in effect lowers the cost of dinner, and everybody likes that.

- Mexican restaurants are not forbidden in the Zone. Chili is a great Zone food. A taco salad is another good choice, or buy a taco plate, eat one of the taco shells, and put the rest of the toppings on a side salad. The same rule applies to fajitas. Eat one tortilla filled with protein and vegetables and then eat all the rest of the toppings. Order corn tortillas instead of flour tortillas. Black beans are also a Zone-favorable carbohydrate. Guacamole is a good choice for monounsaturated fat, but stay away from other high-fat choices.

- We used to get very hungry about an hour after we ate Chinese food in our pre-Zone days. It was the rice that was the culprit. That's a great example of how less starch is more on the Zone Diet. Now we order a healthy Chinese entrée with protein, such as ginger shrimp, chicken and broccoli, or a tofu entrée, and then split another vegetable dish.

- A steakhouse, such as Outback, usually serves outlandishly large protein servings. Imagine eating a 20-ounce porterhouse steak. Instead, Shrimp on the Barbie, a selection of vegetables, the French onion soup, and a glass of wine works just about right. Or try salads topped with chicken or shrimp and sides of grilled onions and sautéed mushrooms. You can also choose the fish of the day, which is lightly seasoned and grilled and served with fresh veggies.

- If you go out for pizza, choose one with a thin crust and a lot of protein. Then enjoy one slice and the toppings of the next piece, leaving the crust behind.

The Omega Zone e-magazine appears monthly on www.drsears.com, and one of the most popular features every month is Sherlock Zone. Sherlock is asked to investigate various national chain restaurants to give diners clues about how to construct a Zone meal, including Applebee's, Bertucci's, and Garcia's, a typical Mexican restaurant. Recently he cracked the case at Panera Bread, whose claim to fame is "fresh-baked bliss." Even though this restaurant is all about bread, Sherlock was able to couple some of the chain's tasty soups with salads. Soups to Sherlock's liking included Black Bean Soup, Farmer's Market Bisque, French Onion, Garden Vegetable, and Vegetable and Sirloin. The black bean is particularly good because it probably contains just about all the carbs you need for your meal. Just don't get your soup served in a bread bowl. Believe me, that won't leave you in a blissful state.

There are a number of salads that can be Zonefully paired with the soup, including Asian Sesame Chicken Salad, Grilled Chicken Caesar Salad, and Fandango Salad. Just don't eat too many croutons. If you want a sandwich, choose one made with thin slices of bread and just eat one slice.

ALCOHOL IN THE ZONE

One time after I gave a talk in Marblehead, Massachusetts, a woman approached me and told me she always has wine with her dinner. I told her to treat alcohol like a carbohydrate. That would mean she would have to have one ounce of protein to have a glass of wine.

"I said I want to have *wine* with dinner," she said.

"How much wine?" I asked.

"Four glasses," she replied.

Well, four glasses of wine with dinner would have most people under the table, but apparently this was her cup of tea. I told her to be rigorous with Zoning her meals for breakfast, lunch, and snacks and to have four ounces of chicken or 6½ ounces of salmon with her four ounces of wine. Please note that four glasses of wine at dinner is definitely not a Zone recommendation, but it was clear that that was what that woman was going to drink at dinner, Zone or no Zone. The beauty of the Zone is its flexibility. By the way, she lost 35 pounds.

—*Barry Sears*

Remember, treat alcohol like a carbohydrate. Before you have one 6-ounce light beer, one 4-ounce glass of wine, or 1 ounce of distilled spirits, you have to have one block of protein. Moderate drinking, obviously, is the goal. If your protein choice is low in fat, have a couple of nuts. Protein examples include:

- 1 ounce lean beef
- 1 ounce skinless turkey or chicken breast
- 1 ounce low-fat cheese
- 1½ ounces of shrimp
- ½ Morningstar Farms Grillers Veggie Burgers
- 1 ounce tuna salad
- 1 ounce ham
- 1½ ounces deli meat

CRUISING IN THE ZONE

Just about every year we are the hosts of a Zone Cruise. Our past cruises have taken us to different parts of the Caribbean, Alaska, and the Mexican Riviera. Highlights include Zone seminars and special meals to help everyone on the cruise stay in the Zone.

Most people who go on cruises, surrounded by the sea and a sea of food, gain a lot of weight. Food is available 24/7. People on a Zone Cruise, on the other hand, lose a pound or two during the week.

Zone staffers are at the buffet in the mornings to help Zone Cruisers learn how to choose a Zone breakfast. At lunch there is the opportunity to either hit the buffet or go to a restaurant where a Zone lunch is served. Gourmet Zone dinners are served every night. Here's one of the dinners served on a Zone Cruise:

APPETIZER

Fresh pineapple gondola

SOUP

Clear oxtail soup

SALAD

Greens, tomato, scallions, and basil Zone dressing

MAIN COURSE

Baked fillet of mahi-mahi served with tomato, bell peppers, onion sauce, and steamed green beans

or

Jerked pork loin marinated with fresh spices and accompanied by grilled tomato and steamed green beans

and

Extra plates of assorted vegetables

DESSERT

Glazed spiced apple

Some of the other desserts served on the cruise, are featured in *Zone-Perfect Meals in Minutes.*

Glazed Spiced Apple

This recipe makes four 1-block servings. It is easy to adjust the blocks up or down depending on how many people you are serving.

Block Size	Ingredients
2 carbohydrate	1 Delicious apple, cored and cut into 1-inch cubes
1 carbohydrate	1 peach, halved, pitted, and finely chopped
½ carbohydrate	1 teaspoon brown sugar
½ carbohydrate	2 teaspoons cornstarch
4 fat	4 teaspoons almonds, sliced and toasted
	⅓ cup water
	3 tablespoons cider vinegar
	¼ teaspoon lemon extract
	⅛ teaspoon ground cinnamon
	Dash celery salt
4 protein	4 ounces low-fat cheddar cheese, shredded (1 cup)

Instructions

In a small saucepan over medium heat, combine all the ingredients except the cheese. Stirring constantly, cook until the apple is thoroughly coated and a sauce forms. Simmer 3 to 5 minutes, or until the flavors are blended. Spoon into bowls, top with shredded cheese, and serve hot.

Even if you don't go on a Zone Cruise, you can still stay in the Zone during a cruise. The buffet offers plenty of low-fat protein choices, fresh fruits, and vegetables. In the restaurants, the servers will be happy to make substitutions.

Life's special occasions usually revolve around food. In the Zone, every day in life is a special occasion—you can eat great-tasting food, lose weight, and be in the best of health.

Now You Can Do It

We hope you can now say, "I can do the Zone." Whether you like to keep your meals simple or enjoy spending time in the kitchen, I hope this book has struck a chord with you. We've given you several different degrees of Zoning. You may stop at any level you want. You may not want to get into learning blocks and grams. That's fine. Use the hand-eye method and put together the combinations laid out for breakfasts, lunches, dinners, and snacks. Remember, the first step the Sears family took was simply to eliminate pasta, potatoes, rice, and French bread and add more vegetables and fruit.

Whatever you do, don't be obsessive about getting it right. Don't anguish if one apple you have is bigger than the other one. Just relax and enjoy yourself as you begin to look better, feel better, and perform better.

As we mentioned in chapter 1, the most important tool for entering and staying in the Zone is a food diary. As you begin the Zone, write down every meal and snack you eat. Then make a note of how you feel four or five hours later. Are you hungry and in a mental fog? Then you had too many carbohydrates at your last meal. Cut back the carbohydrates the next time you eat that exact same meal (by one block, if you're using the Food Block method), but keep the protein and fat sizes the same. On the other hand, if you are hungry and have good mental focus, that means you ate too few carbohydrates at your last meal. When Zoners say they're hungry an hour or two after lunch, we usually correctly guess they had a grilled chicken Caesar salad and nothing else. You have to eat a field of lettuce to get enough carbohydrate blocks. The next time you have that exact same meal, add an apple and a small breadstick. Or do as we did to feed our finicky teen who would only eat green things: take out a bowl of grapes or slice a Granny Smith apple.

Several different styles of cooking are presented in this book. Rachel Albert-Matesz's recipes contain 16 blocks each. That means they provide four 4-block meals, five 3-block meals and a snack, or other combinations, so they're perfect for parties. Many also often contain two different recipes, such as frittata and a smoothie or fruit salad. Diane Manteca's recipes in chapter 8 contain 8 blocks each, just about right for a dinner for two. Choose the style that best suits you.

If you're in the Zone, you'll soon come to realize it's a real physiological state in which you are able to keep the hormone insulin in a range that's not too high and not too low. We hope you will never need to buy another women's magazine just to try the "diet to end all diets." The Zone diet is it! And it's not just a diet. It's an eating plan that you will follow for the rest of your life. When people come up to you and say that they wish they were naturally thin like you, you can do two things—either smile and nod or let them in on your secret.

Appendix A

Continuing Support

Although this book was written to make following the Zone diet incredibly easy, there will always be more questions. That is why we have developed several unique websites to give you that backup support. The portal site to all of the Web sites is www.zonediet.com the official website of the Zone diet. The informative sites you will find at this portal site include www.drsears.com, an all-inclusive site that provides approved recipes, helpful hints, continuing research, daily updates on the latest breaking medical news, and answers to the best questions submitted to the site. Another innovative feature of www.zonediet.com is Zone TV, our Internet-based TV studio, and Zone Radio, on which we host the monthly programs "Living in the Zone" and "Ask the Doctors." On the latter, we interview leading medical researchers about chronic disease conditions and how the Zone diet can have an impact on them. Finally, check out www.drsearszonelabs.com, where you can find the patented products Dr. Sears developed to help keep you in the Zone. Or simply call Zone Labs at 1-800-404-8171 for more information.

Food Block Guide

PROTEIN BLOCKS
(Approximately 7 grams of protein per block)

MEAT AND POULTRY

Best Choices (Low in saturated fat)
Beef (range-fed or game), 1 ounce
Chicken breast, skinless, 1 ounce
Chicken breast, deli-style, 1½ ounces
Turkey breast, skinless, 1 ounce
Turkey breast, deli-style, 1½ ounces
Turkey, ground, 1½ ounces
Turkey bacon, 3 strips
Lean Canadian bacon, 1 ounce
Ground beef (less than 10 percent fat), 1½ ounces

Fair Choices (Moderate in saturated fat)
Beef, lean cuts, 1 ounce
Beef, ground (less than 10 percent fat), 1½ ounces
Canadian bacon, lean, 1 ounce
Chicken, dark meat, skinless, 1 ounce
Corned beef, lean, 1 ounce
Duck, 1½ ounces
Ham, lean, 1 ounce
Ham, deli-style, 1½ ounces

Lamb, lean, 1 ounce
Pork, lean, 1 ounce
Pork chop, 1 ounce
Turkey bacon, 3 slices
Turkey, dark meat, skinless, 1 ounce
Veal, 1 ounce

Poor Choices (High in saturated fat, arachidonic acid, or both)

Bacon, pork, 3½ slices
Beef, fatty cuts,* 1 ounce
Beef, ground (more than 10 percent fat), 1½ ounces
Hot dog, beef or pork, 1 link
Hot dog, chicken or turkey, 1 link
Pepperoni, 1 ounce
Salami, 1 ounce
Sausage, pork, 2 links
Sausage, pork, 2 patties

Fish and Seafood

Bass, freshwater, 1 ounce
Bass, sea, 1½ ounces
Bluefish, 1½ ounces
Calamari, 1½ ounces
Catfish, 1½ ounces
Clams, 1½ ounces
Cod, 1½ ounces
Crabmeat, 1½ ounces
Haddock, 1½ ounces
Halibut, 1½ ounces
Lobster, 1½ ounces
Mackerel, 1½ ounces
Salmon, 1½ ounces
Sardine, 1 ounce
Scallops, 1½ ounces
Shrimp, 1½ ounces
Snapper, 1½ ounces
Swordfish, 1½ ounces

Trout, 1½ ounces
Tuna, steak, 1 ounce
Tuna, canned in water, 1 ounce

EGGS

Best Choices
Egg whites (large), 2
Egg substitute, ¼ cup

Fair Choice
Whole egg,* 1

PROTEIN-RICH DAIRY

Best Choices
Cheese, nonfat, 1 ounce
Cottage cheese, low-fat, ¼ cup

Fair Choices
Cheese, low-fat, 1 ounce
Mozzarella cheese, skim, 1 ounce
Ricotta cheese, skim, 2 ounces

Poor Choices
Hard cheeses, 1 ounce

PROTEIN-RICH VEGETARIAN (Always check package labels)
Tofu, firm or extra firm, 2 ounces
Soy Canadian bacon, 3 slices
Soy sausage, 1 link
Soy hot dog, 1 link
Soy hamburger crumbles, ½ cup
Soy protein powder (7 grams protein), ⅓ ounce
Soy burgers, ½ patty
Soy hot dog, 1 link
Soy sausage, links, 2 links
Soy sausage, patty, 1 patty

*Contains arachidonic acid

MIXED PROTEIN SOURCES
(Contain more carbohydrates, so read labels carefully)
Soybeans, boiled, ¼ block
Soybean hamburger, ¾ patty
Tofu, silken, 5 ounce
Tofu, soft, 4 ounce

PROTEIN/CARBOHYDRATE
(Contains 1 block protein and 1 block carbohydrate)
OmegaZone Nutrition bar, ½ bar
Milk, low-fat (1%), 1 cup
Soy milk, 8 ounce
Soy flour, 10 grams
Yogurt, plain, ½ cup
Tempeh, 1½ ounces

CARBOHYDRATE BLOCKS
(Approximately 9 grams of carbohydrates per block)

LOW-DENSITY CARBOHYDRATES

Cooked Vegetables
Artichoke, 4 large
Artichoke hearts, 1 cup
Asparagus, 1 cup (12 spears)
Beans, green or wax, 1½ cups
Beans, black, ¼ cup
Bok choy, 3 cups
Broccoli, 3 cups
Brussels sprouts, 1½ cups
Cabbage, 3 cups
Cauliflower, 4 cups
Chickpeas, ¼ cup
Collard greens, chopped, 2 cups
Eggplant, 1½ cups
Kale, 2 cups
Kidney beans, ¼ cup

Leeks, 1 cup

Lentils, ¼ cup

Mushrooms, boiled, 2 cups

Okra, sliced, 1 cup

Onions, chopped boiled, ½ cup

Sauerkraut, 1 cup

Spaghetti squash, 1 cup

Swiss chard, chopped, 2½ cups

Turnip, mashed, 1½ cups

Turnip greens, chopped, 4 cups

Yellow (summer) squash, sliced, 2 cups

Zucchini, sliced, 2 cups

Raw Vegetables

Alfalfa sprouts, 10 cups

Bamboo shoots, 4 cups

Bean sprouts, 3 cups

Broccoli, florets, 4 cups

Brussels sprouts, 1½ cups

Cabbage, shredded, 4 cups

Cauliflower, florets, 4 cups

Celery, sliced, 2 cups

Chickpeas, ¼ cup

Cucumber (medium), 1½

Cucumber, sliced, 4 cups

Endive, chopped, 10 cups

Escarole, chopped, 10 cups

Green or red peppers, 2

Green or red pepper, chopped, 2 cups

Hummus, ¼ cup

Jalapeño peppers, 2 cups

Lettuce, iceberg (6-inch diameter), 2 heads

Lettuce, romaine,chopped, 10 cups

Mushrooms, chopped, 4 cups

Onions, chopped, 1½ cups

Radishes, sliced, 4 cups

Salsa, ½ cup

Snow peas, 1½ cups
Spinach, chopped, 10 cups
Spinach salad (3 cups raw spinach, ¾ cup raw onion, and 1 raw tomato), 1
Tomato, 2
Tomato, cherry, 2 cups
Tomato, chopped, 1½ cups
Tossed salad (3 cups shredded lettuce, 1 raw green pepper, and 1 raw tomato)
Water chestnuts, ⅓ cup
Watercress, 10 cups

Fruits (fresh, frozen, or canned light)
Apple, ½
Applesauce, unsweetened, ⅓ cup
Apricots, 3
Blackberries, ¾ cup
Blueberries, ½ cup
Boysenberries, ½ cup
Cherries, 8
Fruit cocktail, light, ⅓ cup
Grapes, ½ cup
Grapefruit, ½
Kiwi, 1
Lemon, 1
Lime, 1
Nectarine, medium, ½
Orange, ½
Orange, Mandarin, canned in water, ⅓ cup
Peach, 1
Peaches, canned in water, ½ cup
Pear, ½
Plum, 1
Raspberries, 1 cup
Strawberries, diced fine, 1 cup
Tangerine, 1

Grains (Read labels)

Barley, dry, ⅛ cup
Oatmeal, slow-cooking, ⅓ cup
Oatmeal, slow-cooking, dry, ½ ounce

HIGH-DENSITY CARBOHYDRATES (Use in moderation)

Cooked Vegetables

Acorn squash, ½ cup
Beans, baked, ¼ cup
Beans, refried, ¼ cup
Beets, sliced, ½ cup
Butternut squash, ½ cup
Carrot, 1
Carrots, sliced, 1 cup
Carrots, shredded, 1 cup
Corn, ¼ cup
French fries, 5
Lima beans, ¼ cup
Parsnips, ⅓ cup
Peas, ½ cup
Pinto beans, ¼ cup
Potato, baked, ¼ cup
Potato, boiled, ⅓ cup
Potato, mashed, ¼ cup
Refried beans, ¼ cup
Sweet potato, baked, ⅓ cup
Sweet potato, mashed, ¼ cup

Fruits

Banana, ⅓
Cantaloupe, ¼ melon
Cantaloupe, cubed, ¾ cup
Cranberries, ¾ cup
Cranberry sauce, 3 teaspoon
Dates, 2 pieces
Fig, 1 piece
Guava, ½ cup

Honeydew melon, cubed, ⅔ cup
Kumquat, 3
Mango, sliced, ⅓ cup
Papaya, cubed, ¾ cup
Pineapple, diced, ½ cup
Prunes, dried, 2
Raisins, 1 tablespoon
Watermelon, cubed, ¾ cup

Fruit Juices
Apple, ⅓ cup
Apple cider, ⅓ cup
Cranberry, ¼ cup
Fruit punch, ¼ cup
Grape, ¼ cup
Grapefruit, ⅓ cup
Lemonade, unsweetened, ⅓ cup
Lime, ⅓ cup
Orange, ⅓ cup
Pineapple, ¼ cup
Tomato, 1 cup
V-8, ¾ cup

Grains, Cereals, and Breads
Bagel, small, ¼
Biscuit, ½
Bread crumbs, ½ ounce
Bread, whole grain or white, ½ slice
Breadstick, hard, 1
Breadstick, soft, ½
Buckwheat, dry, ½ ounce
Bulgur wheat, dry, ½ ounce
Cereal, dry, ½ ounce
Cornbread, 1-inch square
Cornstarch, 4 teaspoons
Couscous, dry, ½ ounce
Cracker, graham, 1½ squares

Cracker, saltine, 4
Cracker, Triscuit, 3
Croissant, plain, ¼
Crouton, ½ ounce
Doughnut, plain, ⅓
English muffin, ¼
Granola, ½ ounce
Grits, cooked, ⅓ cup
Melba toast, ½ ounce
Millet, dry, ½ ounce
Muffin, blueberry, mini, ½
Noodles, egg, cooked, ¼ cup
Pancake, four-inch, 1
Pasta, cooked, ¼ cup
Pita bread, ½ pocket
Pita bread, mini, ⅓ pocket
Popcorn, popped, 2 cups
Rice, brown, cooked, ⅓ cup
Rice, white, cooked, ⅓ cup
Rice cake, 1
Roll, bulkie, ¼
Roll, small dinner, ½
Roll, hamburger, ½
Taco shell, 1
Tortilla, six-inch corn, 1
Tortilla, eight-inch flour, ½
Waffle, ½

Alcohol
Beer, light, 6 ounces or ½ bottle
Beer, regular, 4 ounces or ⅓ bottle
Distilled spirits, 1 ounce
Wine, 4 ounces

Others
Barbecue sauce, 2 tablespoons
Cake, ⅓ slice

Candy bar, ¼
Catsup, 2 tablespoons
Cocktail sauce, 2 tablespoons
Cookie, small, 1
Honey, ½ tablespoon
Ice cream, regular, ¼ cup
Ice cream, premium, ⅙ cup
Jam or jelly, 2 tablespoons
Molasses, light, ½ teaspoon
Plum sauce, 1½ tablespoons
Potato chips, ½ ounce
Pretzels, ½ ounce
Relish, pickle, 4 teaspoons
Sugar, brown, 2 teaspoons
Sugar, granulated, 2 teaspoons
Sugar, confectionary, 1 tablespoon
Syrup, maple, 2 teaspoons
Syrup, pancake, 2 teaspoons
Teriyaki sauce, 1 tablespoon
Tortilla chips, ½ ounce

FAT BLOCKS

(There are approximately 1.5 grams of fat per block; if you are using the gram method and calculating hidden fat, double the fat amount to 3 grams.)

Best Choices (rich in monounsaturated fat)

Almond butter, ½ teaspoon
Almond oil, ⅓ teaspoon
Almond, slivered, 1 teaspoon
Almonds, whole, 3
Avocado, 1 tablespoon
Cashews, 2
Guacamole, 1 tablespoon
Macadamia nuts, 1
Olives, 3

Olive oil, ⅓ teaspoon
Olive oil and vinegar dressing (⅓ teaspoon olive oil plus vinegar to taste)
Peanuts, 6
Peanut oil, ⅓ teaspoon
Peanut butter, natural, ½ teaspoon
Tahini, ½ teaspoon

Fair Choices (Low in saturated fat)

Canola oil, ⅓ teaspoon
Mayonnaise, regular, ⅓ teaspoon
Mayonnaise, light, 1 teaspoon
Sesame oil, ½ teaspoon
Soybean oil, ⅓ teaspoon
Walnuts, shelled and chopped, ½ teaspoon

Poor Choices (Rich in saturated fat)

Bacon bits, imitation, 2 teaspoons
Butter, ⅓ teaspoon
Cream (half and half), ½ tablespoon
Cream cheese, 1 teaspoon
Cream cheese, light, 2 teaspoons
Lard, ⅓ teaspoon
Sour cream, ½ tablespoon
Sour cream, light, 1 tablespoon
Vegetable shortening, ⅓ teaspoon

Calculation of Your Daily Protein Requirements

1. Determine your lean body mass by consulting Appendix D.
2. Determine your activity factor. Factors are listed below in grams of protein per pound of lean body mass.

   0.5 - Sedentary (no formal sports activity or training)
   0.6 - Light fitness training, such as walking
   0.7 - Moderate training (3 times a week) or sports participation
   0.8 - Daily aerobic training or daily moderate weight training
   0.9 - Heavy daily weight training
   1.0 - Heavy daily weight training coupled with intense sports training or twice-a-day intense sports training

3. Finally, calculate your required daily amount of protein (in grams): multiply your lean body mass (in lbs.) by your activity factor.

The following table will give you representative protein requirements based on lean body mass and activity factors.

	ACTIVITY FACTOR (grams of protein per pound of lean body mass)					
Lean Body Mass (in lbs.)	**0.5**	**0.6**	**0.7**	**0.8**	**0.9**	**1.0**
90	45	54	63	72	81	90
100	50	60	70	80	90	100
110	55	66	77	88	99	110
120	60	72	84	96	108	120
130	65	78	91	104	117	130
140	70	84	98	112	126	140
150	75	90	105	120	135	150
160	80	96	112	128	144	160
170	85	102	119	136	153	170
180	90	108	126	144	162	180
190	95	114	133	152	171	190
200	100	120	140	160	180	200
210	105	126	147	168	189	210
220	110	132	154	176	198	220
230	115	138	161	184	207	230
240	120	144	168	192	216	240

Calculation of Percent Body Fat

A rapid way to determine your percent body fat is simply to use a tape measure. You should make all measurements on bare skin (not through clothing), and make sure that the tape fits snugly but does not compress the skin and underlying tissue. Take all measurements three times and calculate the average. All measurements should be in inches.

Calculating Body-Fat Percentages for Females

There are five steps you must take to calculate your percentage of body fat:

1 While keeping the tape level, measure your hips at their widest point, and your waist at the umbilicus (i.e., belly button). It is critical that you measure at the belly button and not at the narrowest point of your waist. Take each of these measurements three times and compute the average.

2 Measure your height in inches without shoes.

3 Record your height, waist, and hip measurements on the accompanying worksheet.

4 Find each of these measurements in the appropriate column in the accompanying tables and record the constants on the worksheet.

5 Add constants A and B, then subtract constant C for this sum and round to the nearest whole number. That figure is your percentage of body fat.

Conversion Constants for Calculation of Percentage of Body Fat in Females

Hips		Abdomen		Height	
Inches	Constant A	Inches	Constant B	Inches	Constant C
30	33.48	20	14.22	55	33.52
30.5	33.83	20.5	14.40	55.5	33.67
31	34.87	21.0	14.93	56	34.13
31.5	35.22	21.5	15.11	56.5	34.28
32	36.27	22	15.64	57	34.74
32.5	36.62	22.5	15.82	57.5	34.89
33	37.67	23	16.35	58	35.35
33.5	38.02	23.5	16.53	58.5	35.50
34	39.06	24	17.06	59	35.96
34.5	39.41	24.5	17.24	59.5	36.11
35	40.46	25	17.78	60	36.57
35.5	40.81	25.5	17.96	60.5	36.72
36	41.86	26	18.49	61	37.18
36.5	42.21	26.5	18.67	61.5	37.33
37	43.25	27	19.20	62	37.79
37.5	43.60	27.5	19.38	62.5	37.94
38	44.65	28	19.91	63	38.40
38.5	45.32	28.5	20.27	63.5	38.70
39	46.05	29	20.62	64	39.01
39.5	46.40	29.5	20.80	64.5	39.16
40	47.44	30	21.33	65	39.62
40.5	47.79	30.5	21.51	65.5	39.77
41	48.84	31	22.04	66	40.23
41.5	49.19	31.5	22.22	66.5	40.38
42	50.24	32	22.75	67	40.84
42.5	50.59	32.5	22.93	67.5	40.99
43	51.64	33	23.46	68	41.45
43.5	51.99	33.5	23.64	68.5	41.60
44	53.03	34	24.18	69	42.06
44.5	53.41	34.5	24.36	69.5	42.21

Hips		Abdomen		Height	
Inches	Constant A	Inches	Constant B	Inches	Constant C
45	54.53	35	24.89	70	42.67
45.5	54.86	35.5	25.07	70.5	42.82
46	55.83	36	25.60	71	43.28
46.5	56.18	36.5	25.78	71.5	43.43
47	57.22	37	26.31	72	43.89
47.5	57.57	37.5	26.49	72.5	44.04
48	58.62	38	27.02	73	44.50
48.5	58.97	38.5	27.20	73.5	44.65
49	60.02	39	27.73	74	45.11
49.5	60.37	39.5	27.91	74.5	45.26
50	61.42	40	28.44	75	45.72
50.5	61.77	40.5	28.62	75.5	45.87
51	62.81	41	29.15	76	46.32
51.5	63.16	41.5	29.33		
52	64.21	42	29.87		
52.5	64.56	42.5	30.05		
53	65.61	43	30.58		
53.5	65.96	43.5	30.76		
54	67.00	44	31.29		
54.5	67.35	44.5	31.47		
55	68.40	45	32.00		
55.5	68.75	45.5	32.18		
56	69.80	46	32.71		
56.5	70.15	46.5	32.89		
57	71.19	47	33.42		
57.5	71.54	47.5	33.60		
58	72.59	48	34.13		
58.5	72.94	48.5	34.31		
59	73.99	49	34.84		
59.5	74.34	49.5	35.02		
60	75.39	50	35.56		

Worksheet for Women to Calculate Their Percentage of Body Fat

Average hip measurement _____ (used for constant A)

Average abdomen measurement _____ (used for constant B)

Height _____ (used for constant C)

Using the table on pages 380 and 381, look up each of the average measurements and your height in the appropriate column.

Constant A = _____

Constant B = _____

Constant C = _____

To determine your approximate percentage of body fat, add constants A and B. From that total, subtract constant C. The result is your percentage of body fat, as shown below.

(Constant A + Constant B) − Constant C = % Body Fat

Calculating Body-Fat Percentages for Men

There are four steps you must take to determine your body-fat percentage:

1. While keeping the tape level, measure the circumference of your waist at the umbilicus (i.e., belly button). Measure three times and compute the average.
2. Measure your wrist at the space between your dominant hand and your wrist bone, at the location where your wrist bends.
3. Record these measurements on the worksheet for men.
4. Subtract your wrist measurement from your waist measurement and find the resulting value listed in the table. On the left-hand side of this table, find your weight. Proceed to the right from your weight and down from your waist-minus-wrist measurement. Where these two points intersect, read your body fat percentage.

Worksheet for Men to Calculate Their Percentage of Body Fat

Average waist measurement _____ (inches)

Average wrist measurement _____ (inches)

Subtract the wrist measurement from the waist measurement. Use the table starting on page 384 to find your weight. Then find your "waist minus wrist" number. Where the two columns intersect is your approximate percentage of body fat.

Male Percentage Body Fat Calculations

Waist-Wrist (in inches)	22	22.5	23	23.5	24
Weight (in pounds)					
120	4	6	8	10	12
125	4	6	7	9	11
130	3	5	7	9	11
135	3	5	7	8	10
140	3	5	6	8	10
145		4	6	7	9
150		4	6	7	9
155		4	5	6	8
160		4	5	6	8
165		3	5	6	8
170		3	4	6	7
175			4	6	7
180			4	5	7
185			4	5	6
190			4	5	6
195			3	5	6
200			3	4	6
205				4	5
210				4	5
215				4	5
220				4	5
225				3	4
230				3	4
235				3	4
240					4
245					4
250					4
255					3
260					3
265					
270					
275					
280					
285					
290					
295					
300					

24.5	25	25.5	26	26.5	27	27.5
14	16	18	20	21	23	25
13	15	17	19	20	22	24
12	14	16	18	20	21	23
12	13	15	17	19	20	22
11	13	15	16	18	19	21
11	12	14	15	17	19	20
10	12	13	15	16	18	19
10	11	13	14	16	17	19
9	11	12	14	15	17	18
9	10	12	13	15	16	17
9	10	11	13	14	15	17
8	10	11	12	12	15	16
8	9	10	12	13	14	16
8	9	10	11	13	14	15
7	8	10	11	12	13	15
7	8	9	11	12	13	14
7	8	9	10	11	12	14
6	8	9	10	11	12	13
6	7	8	9	11	12	13
6	7	8	9	10	11	12
6	7	8	9	10	11	12
6	7	8	9	10	11	12
5	6	7	8	9	10	11
5	6	7	8	9	10	11
5	6	7	8	9	10	11
5	6	7	8	9	9	10
5	6	6	7	8	9	10
4	5	6	7	8	9	10
4	5	6	7	8	9	10
4	5	6	7	8	8	9
4	5	6	7	7	8	9
4	5	5	6	7	8	9
4	4	5	6	7	8	9
4	4	5	6	7	8	8
3	4	5	6	7	7	8
3	4	5	6	6	7	8
3	4	5	5	6	7	8

Waist-Wrist (in inches)	28	28.5	29	29.5	30	30.5	31
Weight (in pounds)							
120	27	29	31	33	35	37	39
125	26	28	30	32	33	35	37
130	25	27	28	30	32	34	36
135	24	26	27	29	31	32	34
140	23	24	26	28	29	31	33
145	22	23	25	27	28	30	31
150	21	23	24	26	27	29	30
155	20	22	23	25	26	28	29
160	19	21	22	24	25	27	28
165	19	20	22	23	24	26	27
170	18	19	21	22	24	25	26
175	17	19	20	21	23	24	25
180	17	18	19	21	22	23	25
185	16	18	19	20	21	23	24
190	16	17	18	19	21	22	23
195	15	16	18	19	20	21	22
200	15	16	17	18	19	21	22
205	14	15	17	18	19	20	21
210	14	15	16	17	18	19	21
215	13	15	16	17	18	19	20
220	13	14	15	16	17	18	19
225	13	14	15	16	17	18	19
230	12	13	14	15	16	17	18
235	12	13	14	15	16	17	18
240	12	13	14	15	16	17	17
245	11	12	13	14	15	16	17
250	11	12	13	14	15	16	17
255	11	12	13	14	14	15	16
260	10	11	12	13	14	15	16
265	10	11	12	13	14	15	15
270	10	11	12	13	13	14	15
275	10	11	11	12	13	14	15
280	9	10	11	12	13	14	14
285	9	10	11	12	12	13	14
290	9	10	11	11	12	13	14
295	9	10	10	11	12	13	14
300	9	9	10	11	12	12	13

31.5	32	32.5	33	33.5	34	34.5
41	43	45	47	49	50	52
39	41	43	45	46	48	50
37	39	41	43	44	46	48
36	38	39	41	43	44	46
34	36	38	39	41	43	44
33	35	36	38	39	41	43
32	33	35	36	38	40	41
31	32	34	35	37	38	40
30	31	33	34	35	37	38
29	30	31	33	34	36	37
28	29	30	32	33	34	36
27	28	29	31	32	33	35
26	27	28	30	31	32	34
25	26	28	29	30	31	33
24	26	27	28	29	30	32
24	25	26	27	28	30	31
23	24	25	26	28	29	30
22	23	25	26	27	28	29
22	23	24	25	26	27	28
21	22	23	24	25	26	28
20	22	23	24	25	26	27
20	21	22	23	24	25	26
19	20	21	22	23	24	25
19	20	21	22	23	24	25
18	19	20	21	22	23	24
18	19	20	21	22	23	24
18	18	19	20	21	22	23
17	18	19	20	21	22	23
17	18	19	19	20	21	22
16	17	18	19	20	21	22
16	17	18	19	19	20	21
16	16	17	18	19	20	21
15	16	17	18	19	19	20
15	16	17	17	18	19	20
15	15	16	17	18	19	19
14	15	16	17	17	18	19
14	15	16	16	17	18	19

Waist-Wrist (in inches)	35	35.5	36	36.5	37
Weight (in pounds)					
120	54				
125	52	54			
130	50	52	53	55	
135	48	50	51	53	55
140	46	48	49	51	53
145	44	46	47	49	51
150	43	44	46	47	49
155	41	43	44	46	47
160	40	41	43	44	46
165	38	40	41	43	44
170	37	39	40	41	43
175	36	37	39	40	41
180	35	36	37	39	40
185	34	35	36	38	39
190	33	34	35	37	38
195	32	33	34	35	37
200	31	32	33	35	36
205	30	31	32	34	35
210	29	30	32	33	34
215	29	30	31	32	33
220	28	29	30	31	32
225	27	28	29	30	31
230	26	27	28	30	31
235	26	27	28	29	30
240	25	26	27	28	29
245	25	26	27	27	28
250	24	25	26	27	28
255	24	24	25	26	27
260	23	24	25	26	27
265	22	23	24	25	26
270	22	23	24	25	25
275	22	22	23	24	25
280	21	22	23	24	24
285	21	21	22	23	24
290	20	21	22	23	23
295	20	21	21	22	23
300	19	20	21	22	22

37.5	38	38.5	39	39.5	40	40.5
54						
52	54	55				
50	52	53	55			
49	50	52	53	55		
47	48	50	51	53	54	
45	47	48	50	51	52	54
44	45	47	48	49	51	52
43	44	45	47	48	49	51
41	43	44	45	47	48	49
40	41	43	44	45	46	48
39	40	41	43	44	45	46
38	39	40	41	43	44	45
37	38	39	40	41	43	44
36	37	38	39	40	41	43
35	36	37	38	39	40	42
34	35	36	37	38	39	40
33	34	35	36	37	38	39
32	33	34	35	36	37	38
32	33	34	35	36	37	38
31	32	33	34	35	36	37
30	31	32	33	34	35	36
29	30	31	32	33	34	35
29	30	31	31	32	33	34
28	29	30	31	32	33	34
27	28	29	30	31	32	33
27	28	29	29	30	31	32
26	27	28	29	30	31	31
26	27	27	28	29	30	31
25	26	27	28	29	29	30
25	26	26	27	28	29	30
24	25	26	27	27	28	29
24	25	25	26	27	28	28
23	24	25	26	26	27	28

Waist-Wrist (in inches)	41	41.5	42	42.5	43	43.5
Weight (in pounds)						
120						
125						
130						
135						
140						
145						
150						
155						
160						
165	55					
170	54	55				
175	52	53	55			
180	50	52	53	54		
185	49	50	51	53	54	55
190	48	49	50	51	52	54
195	46	47	49	50	51	52
200	45	46	47	48	50	51
205	44	45	46	47	48	49
210	43	44	45	46	47	48
215	42	43	44	45	46	47
220	41	42	43	44	45	46
225	40	41	42	43	44	45
230	39	40	41	42	44	44
235	38	39	40	41	42	43
240	37	38	39	40	41	42
245	36	37	38	39	40	41
250	35	36	37	38	39	40
255	34	35	36	37	38	39
260	34	35	35	36	37	38
265	33	34	35	36	36	37
270	32	33	34	35	36	37
275	32	32	33	34	35	36
280	31	32	33	33	34	35
285	30	31	32	33	34	34
290	30	31	31	32	33	34
295	29	30	31	32	32	33
300	29	29	30	31	32	33

44	44.5	45	45.5	46	46.5	47
55						
53	55					
52	53	54	55			
51	52	53	54	55		
49	50	51	53	54	55	
48	49	50	51	52	53	54
47	48	49	50	51	52	53
46	47	48	49	50	51	52
45	46	47	48	49	50	51
44	45	46	47	48	49	50
43	44	45	46	46	47	48
42	43	44	44	45	46	47
41	42	43	44	44	45	46
40	41	42	43	44	44	45
39	40	41	42	43	43	44
38	39	40	41	42	43	43
37	38	39	40	41	42	43
37	38	38	39	40	41	42
36	37	38	38	39	40	41
35	36	37	38	39	39	40
35	35	36	37	38	39	39
34	35	36	36	37	38	39
33	34	35	36	36	37	38

Waist-Wrist (in inches)	47.5	48	48.5	49	49.5	50
Weight (in pounds)						
120						
125						
130						
135						
140						
145						
150						
155						
160						
165						
170						
175						
180						
185						
190						
195						
200						
205						
210						
215	55					
220	54	55				
225	53	54	55			
230	52	53	54	55		
235	51	51	52	53	54	55
240	49	50	51	52	53	54
245	48	49	50	51	52	53
250	47	48	49	50	51	52
255	46	47	48	49	50	51
260	45	46	47	48	49	50
265	44	45	46	47	48	49
270	43	44	45	46	47	48
275	43	43	44	45	46	47
280	42	43	43	44	45	46
285	41	42	43	43	44	45
290	40	41	42	43	43	44
295	39	40	41	42	43	43
300	39	39	40	41	42	43

Index